Praise for Cal Orey and *The Healing Powers of Coffee*

"A cup or two of joe every day is a good way to boost mood, energy and overall health."

—Julian Whitaker, M.D., founder of the
Whitaker Wellness Institute

"For heart, mind, and body, Cal Orey shows us why coffee is the most comforting health food on the planet."

—Will Clower, Ph.D., founder and president
of Mediterranean Wellness, Inc.

"Can coffee be a fountain of youth? Yes! This book can help you add years to your life."

—Karlis Ullis, M.D., Medical Director of Sports Medicine &
Preventative Medical Group, Santa Monica, California

"Cal Orey delivers a tour de force in coffee culture revealing the health benefits and discovering new trends like Single-Serve Coffee Pods along the way. She does all the work so you can reap the benefits."

—"Miss Ellie" Glidewell, Coffee.org

"All of the Healing Powers books have been widely popular on our network of thousands of food bloggers. Her latest book on coffee is no exception!"

—Jenn Campus, Foodie Blogroll

"Cal Orey's in-depth research of all things coffee may be her best book yet—full of great tips, info and history that make you smell the aroma of hot java!"

—Denise Cassino, Long Story Short Newsletter

"The fact that *The Healing Powers of Coffee* was written by Cal Orey is—to coin a phrase—grounds enough to read it. Like a fine cup of that magical potion, this book is to be tasted, appreciated, enjoyed. If you're already a fan of Cal's, you already know her writing is fascinating, personal, scientifically precise and practical. If you enjoy coffee and its mystique, you *must* read this book and you'll appreciate coffee even more!"

—Jonathan M. Purver, *Tahoe Daily Tribune*

The Healing Powers of

Coffee

A Complete Guide to Nature's Surprising Superfood

CAL OREY

KENSINGTON BOOKS
www.kensingtonbooks.com

Permission to reproduce The Mediterranean Diet Pyramid and Common Foods and Flavors of the Mediterranean Diet Pyramid © 2009, granted by Oldways Preservation & Exchange Trust, www.oldwayspt.org

KENSINGTON BOOKS are published by

Kensington Publishing Corp.
119 West 40th Street
New York, NY 10018

All Kensington titles, imprints, and distributed lines are available at special quantity discounts for bulk purchases for sales promotion, premiums, fundraising, educational, or institutional use.

Special book excerpts or customized printings can also be created to fit specific needs. For details, write or phone the office of the Kensington Special Sales Manager: Kensington Publishing Corp., 119 West 40th Street, New York, NY 10018. Attn. Special Sales Department. Phone: 1-800-221-2647.

Kensington and the K logo Reg. U.S. Pat. & TM Off.

ISBN-13: 978-0-7582-7330-7
ISBN-10: 0-7582-7330-4

First Kensington Trade Paperback Printing: August 2012
10 9 8 7 6 5 4

Printed in the United States of America

This book is not intended to replace medical advice. Be sure to consult a physician before adding coffee to your diet.

This book is dedicated to the remarkable coffee tree. I feel an uncanny connection to trees with a purpose—a constant work of nature. The end result: healthful surprises to mankind around the globe.

CONTENTS

Foreword

In writing the Foreword to *The Healing Powers of Coffee*, I am confronted by the delicious ubiquity of this most friendly of drinks. For hundreds of years, coffee has started our day, ended our meals, and served as nucleation for budding conversations in cafés around the globe. And today, its recent retail explosion penetrates our cultural awareness to a degree that we have not seen previously in our lifetimes.

What a perfect time for this book! What a perfect time to take a fresh look at the eye-opening health properties of coffee. There are some myths to overcome, new data to consider, and an even stronger array of reasons to wrap two hands around this beverage and make it part of your daily routine.

COFFEE, THE TIMELESS

Coffee has become that anchor of sanity that brings in the morning for over 150 million Americans every day. And even though it has morphed over time from a "cup of joe" steaming from the curved ceramic mug of the local diner to a specialty drink made from specialty cafes, the essence of coffee's ritual comfort remains. For our parents and their parents, this delicious drink has been a red thread of cultural continuity across time.

Even today, coffee remains woven so completely into the folds of our everyday experience that it carries the comfortable feeling of your favorite jeans that bring recurrent pleasure with each new wearing. At my own house, for example, we have "couch time" every morning, where our own ritual has me making the coffee at 6:00 A.M. My wife and I share that drink together on the couch for 20 minutes every single morning, before wading into the Class-5 rapids of another day. Like millions of other experiences—all similar but different—our daily coffee couch time conversation becomes a continuity of our enduring relationship with coffee.

COFFEE, OUR RITUAL BEVERAGE

While living in France for two years, doing research on the brain, I went through the wonderful routine of eating lunch every day. There are many misconceptions about the relaxed pace of eating in this part of the world. For example, although it's true that their lunch period is actually more of a lunch epoch, lingering on until about 2:30 every day, they are not eating the entire time. It actually takes them about 40 minutes or so to finish their meal.

This is where ritual comes in. After every lunch, we would amble off to "finish" the meal with a little espresso. The point wasn't to bring a lidded, big-gulp bucket of what is essentially a caffeine delivery device back to your desk, but to sit with your friends and talk over this lovely beverage. Within this daily ritual, coffee is a product but, more important, a process of communicating with people.

COFFEE, THE HEALTH DRINK

The Mediterranean people have one of the healthiest diets on earth, and they drink coffee every day. It's funny, though, because when I suggest to people that we should follow suit and add a cup of coffee to our lives, I'm often met with shrieks of protest or dismay. People with those concerns, however, need to "wake up and smell the coffee," because the most recent data confirms what you see in healthy cultures around the planet: Our favorite common morning eye-opener is extremely good for you.

I know, I know. Coffee was associated with cancer some 60 years ago, but according to newer massive studies, coffee consumption is associated with decreased risk of cancer (colon, breast, and prostate). So, if you're concerned about the kinds of foods you need to eat in order to prevent the development of those cancers, you may just want to sit down, have a cup of coffee, and mull it over.

While you're thinking over the internal organs you're protecting with your java jolt, keep in mind that you're also doing your brain a favor. Coffee consumption also improves cognitive function, so you think better. And at the risk of sounding like a late-night infomercial (But Wait There's More!), it is also associated with a reduced risk of Parkinson's as well as Alzheimer's disease. So don't forget to take your coffee in the morning or you may start forgetting to take your coffee in the morning.

COFFEE, TO LOVE

All those incredible health properties of coffee are available when you have it in control. If you have a couple or three cups per day, you get all that brain boosting and cancer prevention. But coffee is like any other food: If a little is healthy for you, a bucket is awful. In other words, the health or ill health of this drink is about not only the coffee itself but also whether you use it or abuse it.

How much is enough/too much? If you need a rule, try this: Love your coffee. Just remember that love is not the same thing as consumption—whether for your food or your drink or anything in your life. The only way to really love your coffee, and get the maximum health benefits from this wonderful drink, is to taste it. Enjoy it. Focus on the flavor, and trade in high-quantity for high-quality consumption. Crazy, right?

It turns out that if you love your coffee in this way, you end up developing a taste for it without needing the sugars or other additives. Even better, when you actually love your coffee and take time with it, you end up controlling consumption through your better behavior. That way, you get to enjoy all the wonderful benefits that Cal Orey's *The Healing Powers of Coffee* reveals, every day.

—Will Clower, Ph.D., author of *The Fat Fallacy: Applying the French Diet to the American Lifestyle* and *The French Don't Diet Plan: 10 Simple Steps to Stay Thin for Life*

Preface

One snowy winter morning, I followed my everyday ritual. I entered the kitchen and brewed a cup of steaming hot coffee. While Mr. Coffee did its job, I fed my Brittany duo and let them outdoors. Then, I poured French Vanilla Roast into a 12-ounce white mug and embraced it, bringing the java back to bed with me. My daily coffee fix is like connecting with a forever friend: reliable, exciting, comforting— always there for me.

After a sip or two of java juice, I tuned in to CNN and retrieved my e-mail. On this particular day, I got an idea. (It's true. Coffee boosts brainpower and the creative process.) I e-mailed my book editor. My words were short and sweet: "Just thinking a tea book to go with the honey book seems like it would work well. What do you think?" His quick response: "Actually, I was thinking of a coffee book since coffee gets a bad rap. Is that a crazy idea?" I typed a one-line answer and clicked *send*. "Not at all. It was my second choice." Like one coffee tree seed, this was the beginning of creating a book on coffee.

During the creation of *The Healing Powers of Chocolate*, I included a chapter titled "A Cuppa Coffee and Chocolat." So, I wasn't a stranger to coffee and its virtues, past and present-day. A while later I sent a follow-up e-mail to my editor. Blame it on the coffee and its caffeine, proven to increase alertness.

"Coffee may be hotter than tea and deserves attention," I noted, and continued on as if I were creating the back cover of a book in progress. "Studies show it can help lower the risk of heart disease, cancer, diabetes; help reduce body fat and unwanted body weight—and increase longevity. Plus, coffee is used in health spa treatments and dozens of home cures and recipes. In moderation, coffee is another superfood and is teamed in cooking/baking with vinegar, olive oil, chocolate, and honey."

As a West Coast native I felt a connection to the potential book topic. After all, I grew up during the Bohemian Beatnik era, which hit the San Francisco Bay Area, where I lived; and in Seattle, Washington, a place where the coffee giant Starbucks originated, growing into a trend that swept the nation and world. These days, coffee, a new health food, is popular for its multitude of coffee roasts, flavored coffees, organic coffee, specialty coffee drinks—hot and cold—and so much more.

It was no surprise that by mid-March the news arrived. The idea of writing a book about coffee and health had come full circle. While I was enjoying my morning cup of Starbucks' Sumatra coffee I was notified by my editor, Richard Ember, that *The Healing Powers of Coffee* was to be my fifth Healing Powers book. I celebrated with a second cup of java juice.

Like vinegar, olive oil, chocolate, and honey, coffee is derived from nature. All five superfoods contain powerful antioxidants and boast versatile uses. The fascinating thing about my journey into the wide world of coffee is that I discovered that coffee is the second most popular commodity in the world.

So like a coffee tree, I began to flourish. The exciting part of my journey is that I discovered that coffee is more than just a beverage to wake up to in the morning. This time around, I'm enjoying a Kona coffee, a slice of gourmet coffee cake, and I just finished a coffee facial. In *The Healing Powers of Coffee* I'll show you how and why this natural beverage from tree to cup will open your eyes to the amazing powers of the coffee tree and its treasures to make your life more complete.

Acknowledgments

Like a coffee tree, during my formative years, teens, and adulthood, it took a while for me to reach maturity. I was a late bloomer as a girl, woman, student—and coffee lover. During the fifties, sixties, seventies, eighties, nineties, and into the 21st century, coffee played a role in my life, bit by bit, like getting to know and love a best friend for life.

Today, as an author, I would like to express my gratitude to the National Coffee Association of U.S.A., Inc., coffee roasters and retailers, my publisher at Kensington, and my editor, Richard Ember, who has guided me through the *Healing Powers* series and who gave me the go-ahead to share the plethora of reasons why the wide world of java deserves a toast.

It's also the coffee trees, from bean to cup, and coffee workers that I will forever be grateful to for their fortitude, past, present, and future. Not to forget hardworking coffee workers and scientists who are on the beat to help keep coffee percolating around the world.

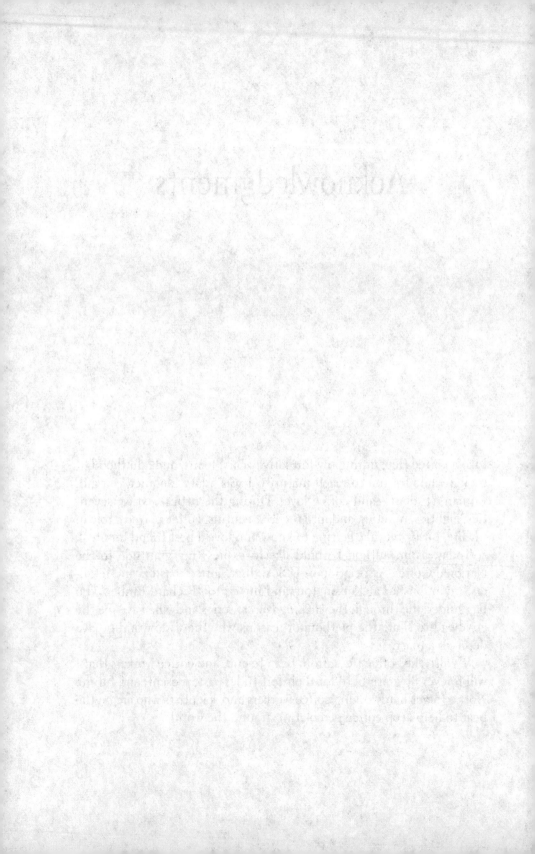

PART 1

A TIME FOR COFFEE

The Power of Coffee

*Ah! How sweet coffee tastes! Lovelier than a thou-
sand kisses, sweeter far than muscatel wine!*
—J. S. Bach, "Coffee Cantata"[1]

More than half a century ago, I was born in a Brazilian villa sitting upon a lush green coffee tree plantation. My mother and father were third-generation migrant coffee roasters. So, I grew up in an atmosphere of a tropical delight. Playing amid the magic of coffee trees with white flowers, red berries, and green beans to cups of java was part of my Coffee World. My father, Jack, from Italy, was a hard worker out in the field overseeing the coffee workers; and my mother, Patricia, with Spanish roots, ran a charming coffee café. That is my fantasy.

In the real world as a little girl (with a big imagination) I didn't live in Brazil, nor was I raised surrounded by coffee trees (actually an evergreen shrub or plant). Back in the fifties, I was born in a suburban neighborhood in San Jose, California—a place where coffee was bought in a can at the store and percolated in an electric coffeepot. My life as I knew it was simple amid houses with white picket fences, sidewalks, and planted shrubs and flowers. It came with two parents—my father was Scottish, my mother Irish Catholic—two siblings, a dog and cat, and the music of the ice-cream man and milk bottles delivered on our doorstep. In our house there was a European-style round table, wall oven, dishwasher, and salmon-colored countertops. I was familiar with the aluminum coffeepot—a constant in my parents' world. It created a strong, familiar coffee aroma wafting into my bedroom seven days a week, including Sundays, the day I went to church.

One fall day, during the priest's sermon, I, a seven-year-old kid, was desperately trying to stay awake. My mother whispered, "Sit up," and nudged my arm. The words "ice cream" were my mantra to help pass the grueling prayers in Latin. After Holy Communion we were released and my mom treated me and my siblings to a local ice-cream parlor.

She ordered a large cup of hot, black coffee (not the kind she served to our priest when he came to dinner). My first coffee experience was in the form of ice cream. Since it was a flavor for grown-ups, I felt like I was entering the land of forbidden fruit. The cold, creamy coffee ice cream was bittersweet. The flavor intrigued me. My taste buds didn't love it; in my mind I liked it. This event began a Sunday ritual. I was hooked on coffee ice cream (maybe it was the caffeine), which ignited my journey into Coffee World.

These days, coffee has a place in my grown-up life as I know it. I wasn't raised on a coffee plantation, but coffee did have a way of permeating its way into my run-of-the-mill life in suburbia—a place where it looked perfect but it was a place from which I yearned to escape to an exciting world. And I got a taste of coffee and its healing powers throughout the years of growing up and blossoming like a young coffee plant with potential to branch out and away from its farm.

Today, I sit here in my mountain cabin, like a coffee tree on a high mountain elevation, and I feel the spirit of the fruitful plant as I work on *The Healing Powers of Coffee*. My kitchen is chock-full of coffees—all kinds—as I scrutinize each one like it is a new, exotic fish in an aquarium. I am discovering the powers of coffee, and a world I've called Coffee World that I want to share with you.

JAVA JOLT: NATURE'S SURPRISE

As legend has it, nature's amazing coffee tree—a member of the Rubiaceae family (genus Coffea)—was first discovered in Ethiopia. Its magical healing powers made eyes open up in Arabia. Then, coffee via man made its journey from country to country, including Turkey, North Africa, and Persia, southern India, and the Balkan states, into Europe, and eventually the United States. As time passed, coffee had made its place throughout the world. And nature's miracle brew continues to surprise people with its plethora of healing virtues.

The first coffee bean (among Turkish rugs and silks) was noted in 1615 in the trade center of Venice. When Pope Clement VIII tasted the coffee, he described it as "heavenly." This declaration upset Italian Christian leaders who claimed it to be "satanic." So, the devil's brew continued to make a controversial presence from the past into even the present day.[2]

Meanwhile, coffee lovers can and do enjoy a variety of coffee beverages—from a simple mug of American roast and espresso-based drinks, such as a cappuccino or latte enriched with milk, to flavored coffees and special blends from regions around the world.

> *Coffee: a beverage made by percolation, infusion, or decoction from the roasted and ground seeds of a coffee plant.*
> —Merriam-Webster's Collegiate Dictionary, 11th edition

COFFEE PLANTS IN A BEAN SHELL

Welcome to the coffee plant, a member of the Rubiaceae family (genus Coffea). Technically speaking, the three most popular species of coffee grown commercially are arabica, robusta, and liberica (similar to robusta). Coffee drinkers, about 75 percent, take to arabica, which is mild, aromatic, and has less caffeine than robusta. The other 25 percent drink robusta (not as high quality as arabica), which is intense and bitter tasting but boasts more caffeine power. Its main use is for its role in tasty coffee blends, espresso, and instant coffees that we turn to for convenience.[3]

Within the genus, the National Coffee Association of U.S.A., Inc., notes the fact that there are over 500 genera and a whopping 6,000 species of tropical trees and shrubs; and coffee plants can range from small shrubs to tall trees, which grow around the globe.

From Seed to Cup

Imagine this scenario: High on a lush, steep hillside frosted with coffee trees, a seasoned picker carries a heavy bag filled with a long day's work and ripe, red coffee cherries. Months from now, the beans from that day's harvest might be the ones in a small bag that you purchase at your favorite store. Between the time he picked them and the time you buy them, the beans went through a series of painstaking steps very much like this:

1. Planting: Did you know a coffee bean is actually a seed? When dried, roasted, and ground, it is used to brew a cup of joe. But if the seed is not processed, it can be planted and will grow into a coffee tree.

2. Harvesting the Cherries: Depending on the variety, it will take about three or four years for the newly planted coffee trees to begin to bear fruit. Whether picked by hand or by machine all coffee is harvested in one of two ways: Strip Picked or Selectively Picked.

3. Processing the Cherries: Once the coffee has been picked, processing begins ASAP, to prevent spoilage, using the dry method (the age-old method used in many countries where water resources are limited) or the wet method. . . .

4. Drying the Beans: If the beans have been processed by the wet method, the pulped and fermented beans must be dried. Once dried, these beans, referred to as "parchment coffee," are warehoused in sisal or jute bags until they are ready for export.

5. Milling the Beans: Before it is exported, coffee is processed by Hulling; Polishing; Grading and Sorting. In many countries, this process is done both by machine and hand, ensuring that only the finest-quality coffee beans are chosen to be exported.

6. Exporting the Beans: The milled beans, now tagged "green coffee," are ready to be loaded onto ships for transport to the importing country. Approximately 7 million tons of green coffee are produced worldwide each year.

7. Tasting the Coffee: Next comes a process known as "cupping" (much like when experts taste olive oil), which takes place in a room designed for the process.

8. Roasting the Coffee: Then, roasting transforms green coffee into the aromatic brown beans that we buy, either whole or already ground, in our favorite stores.

9. Grinding Coffee: The objective of a proper grind (by using a blade or preferred mill grinder to get an even powder) is to get the most flavor in a cup of coffee.

10. Brewing Coffee: So, that's the story in a coffee bean shell about the way coffee beans have traveled to your kitchen. (For more information, refer to chapter 15 "Specialty Coffee Connoisseurs.")

(*Courtesy:* National Coffee Association of U.S.A., Inc.)

MAKING THE GRADE OF COFFEE

Brewing coffee, like harvesting its trees, is a learned art, and knowing the grades of coffee, like chocolate, can help you to grade your cup of java's quality, which varies by country, bean size, bean density, defects, growing altitude, and taste. Here are some decoded "grades" to help you get a handle on terms so you'll understand what's inside a coffee bag.[4]

AA: Refers to a specific, larger than normal bean size. AA+ refers to coffee beans AA or larger. The term AA is used as a coffee quality grade, which can vary from coffee bean size and flavor.

Altura: Means "height" in Spanish and is used to describe high-grown, or mountain-grown, coffee.

Excelso: Used mostly in grading Colombian coffee. Excelso beans are large, but a bit smaller than Supremo coffee beans.

Hard/Strictly Bean: Refers to coffee grown at altitudes 4,000 to 4,500 feet above sea level. The taste of high-grown beans makes them more desirable and expensive than coffees grown at lower elevations.

Strictly Hard Bean: Coffee grown at altitudes higher than 4,500 feet above sea level.

Supremo: Used mostly as a coffee-grading term in Colombia. Supremo coffee beans are slightly larger than Excelso beans.

A TASTE OF FOUR ROASTS

While the process of seed to cup is time consuming, it doesn't go unappreciated. Like more than 50 percent of American households, you may have coffee in your kitchen cupboard but can't tell the difference between a light and dark roast.

There are four basic color categories—light, medium, medium-dark, and dark—for both your health and taste. A debate continues between scientists about whether dark or medium roast contains the most antioxidant power. (For more light on this topic, refer to chapter 4, "Where Are the Secret Ingredients?")

Roast	Description of Coffee	Varieties
Light Roasts	light brown in color; milder coffee	Light City, Half City, Cinnamon, New England
Medium Roasts	medium brown in color with a stronger flavor	City, American, Breakfast
Medium-Dark Roasts	rich, dark color with a slight bittersweet aftertaste	Full City
Dark Roasts	a pronounced bitterness; the darker the roast, the less acidity will be found in the coffee beverage	High, Continental, New Orleans, European, Viennese, Italian, French

(*Courtesy:* National Coffee Association of U.S.A., Inc.)

THE HEALTH BUZZ ABOUT JOE

Not only are there different roasts of coffee to savor, but there are a wide variety of blends and different ways to prepare it. Coffees put to use solo or in drinks are making the news around the world and are in demand from fast-food drive-thrus to five-star restaurants, health spas, beauty salons, businesses, and coffeehouses. (Refer to chapter 2, "An Awakening of Java.")

Coffee is not just a beverage to wake you up in the morning or help you pull an all-nighter at college or work. It's an ancient medicine that has finally been getting kudos from the medical world because it may help lower the risk of developing conditions from heart disease to cancers and diabetes and even prevent conditions from gallstones to dental caries. Coffee is also touted to help stoke your metabolism, which can help take off unwanted pounds and body fat.

Top scientists and medical doctors know coffee health studies show this superfood contains the same—and even more—disease-fighting antioxidant compounds that are found in fruits and vegetables, which fight heart disease, cancers, diabetes, and obesity, four problems in the United States and around the globe.

Drs. Sanjiv Chopra and Alan Lotvin, authors of *Doctor Chopra Says: Medical Facts and Myths Everyone Should Know,* discuss coffee and call it a "lifesaver": "If you're like most people, coffee can be very beneficial for you. And more coffee is even better for you. Coffee has been shown to reduce the incidence of several serious diseases."[5]

Jonny Bowden, Ph.D., renowned author of *The 150 Healthiest Foods on Earth: The Surprising, Unbiased Truth About What You Should Eat and Why,* also praises coffee in his book: "If you're surprised to find coffee on the list of the world's healthiest foods, you're not alone. But when coffee showed up on a couple of my experts' top ten lists, I started really looking at the research and quickly realized that coffee was actually pretty darn good for you."[6]

While most people enjoy a coffee for its jolt of caffeine power, which acts as a stimulant, back in 2005, chemistry professor Joe A. Vinson, Ph.D., and his team of researchers at the University of Scranton, Pennsylvania, analyzed the antioxidant content of dozens of foods, including vegetables, fruits, nuts, spices, and oils. They found that coffee is the number one source of antioxidants in the U.S. diet. And this mind-blowing discovery is just one sobering finding of coffee's perks.

Most medical doctors and nutritionists I spoke with are aware of the healthful compounds in coffee. Yet, while coffee is not 100 percent perfect, its "good food" reputation keeps on percolating in the science world and outweighs the "bad food" rap.

Health-Boosting Nutrients in Coffee

Medical researchers around the world continue to find new health-promoting supernutrients in coffee connected to healing powers. That's right: Coffee lovers are getting more than just a morning caffeine jolt from the magical bean. Like dark chocolate, red wine, green tea, and certain fruits and vegetables, coffee contains antioxidants— disease-fighting enzymes that protect your body by trapping free-radical molecules. Imagine this scenario: Video game human java junkies drinking cups of coffee and viewing bad bugs disappear before any damage attacks their human bodies. Game over. Man wins.

Research also shows that including antioxidant-rich superfoods—like coffee—may lower the risk of developing age-related diseases and even stall the aging process. Researchers continue to find new health-promoting nutrients in coffee—which has more than 1,000 compounds. It's the antioxidants in coffee that provide health benefits; however, coffee also has health-boosting minerals, such as tocopherols and magnesium, which help in glucose metabolism. Here are several antioxidants that researchers know are in a cup of coffee and coffee lovers should meet before I expound later on their benefits to lower the odds of developing specific diseases and ailments:

Caffeic acid: one of the most powerful antioxidants linked to coffee's good-for-you benefits
Chlorogenic acid: like caffeic acid, another potent antioxidant and touted in health studies
Flavonoids: a group of plant compounds that boast antioxidant, anticancer, and antiallergy properties
Lignans: plant compounds with protective action against cancers, especially hormone related, like breast and prostate cancers

Polyphenols: natural compounds that act as powerful antioxidants that protect your body by trapping the free-radical molecules and getting rid of them before damage occurs

Proanthocyanidins: plant compounds helpful in preventing degenerative disease; powerful antioxidants that are stronger than vitamins C and E; help protect against the effects of environmental stressors, including cigarette smoking, pollution

Trigonelline: another antioxidant in coffee, which is linked to aroma, taste, and antibacterial properties

THE COFFEE LOVER'S LEXICON

Here are some other familiar coffee-related words that come up often in Coffee World and I'd like to introduce you to each one—and you'll get to know them better in upcoming chapters.

Term to Know	Definition	The Real Deal
Caffeine	The chemical in coffee that creates a stimulating effect in the human brain and nervous system	Some health pros and cons
Decaffeinated	Coffee with at least 97 percent of its original caffeine content removed	Some health benefits
Gourmet Coffee	Sometimes called special or premium coffee, gourmet coffees made from Arabica beans grown in ideal coffee-producing climates, harvested by hand	It's the crème of the crop
Fair Trade	Fair market wages and working conditions by producers	Fair market prices and habitats to coffee farmers

Organic	Coffee beans that haven't been sprayed with pesticides	Trees taken care of to enrich the forest
Green Coffee	Raw beans	Retain freshness
Single-Origin	Unblended coffee from a single geographical location (e.g., estate coffees)	Provides a distinct flavor
Whole Bean	Ungrounded coffee bean	Has the advantage of staying fresh much longer than ground coffee

EYE-OPENING COFFEE TIDBITS

Since the process of bean to cup goes through an amazing experience to give mankind coffee's healing powers, it makes sense to provide some eye-opening coffee facts revealing its wow factor. Take a look at these fascinating factoids that'll show you its strong jolt of power around the globe.

1. Coffee is the second-most-traded product in the world (after petroleum).
2. Brazil, the world's largest coffee-producing nation, is responsible for 30 to 40 percent of the total world output.
3. It takes five years for a coffee tree to reach maturity. The average annual yield from one tree is the equivalent of one pound of roasted coffee.
4. Twenty-seven percent of U.S. coffee drinkers add a sweetener to their coffee. This compares to 43 percent of German drinkers who add a sweetener.
5. Thirty-five percent of coffee drinkers prefer black coffee; 65 percent prefer to add cream and/or sugar.
6. Women say that drinking coffee "is a good way to relax," while men indicate that coffee "helps them get the job done."
7. Coffee beans are actually berries. Coffee's botanical classification as a fruit helps explain its high level of health antioxidants.
8. All coffee is grown within 1,000 miles of the equator, from the

Tropic of Cancer in the north to the Tropic of Capricorn in the south.

9. To make a roasted pound of coffee it takes around 2,000 hand-picked Arabica coffee cherries. With two beans per cherry, this means around 4,000 beans are in a single pound of coffee.

10. Coffee grows in more than 50 countries, and Hawaii is the only coffee-producing state.

(*Courtesy:* The Oldways Conference on Refreshingly Good News for Coffee Lovers, New York, NY 2006; The Roast and Post Coffee Company; real coffee.co.uk.)

It's not rocket science to get that your favorite coffee, from tree to cup, is part of a painstaking process and deserves its ranking as a prized commodity—and a superfood (a food that provides health benefits) for people like you and me.

Here is a recipe that is both healthful and energizing and you can brew it without the help of a barista. Then, sit back and sip your beverage as you come with me back into ancient times and a present-day exciting Jurassic Park type of Coffee World that'll wow you and keep you on edge with its giant surprises.

Seize the Day Café au Lait

❖ ❖ ❖

⅔ cup low-fat (2 percent) milk
2 teaspoons chocolate-flavored syrup
⅛ teaspoon almond extract
⅔ cup hot, brewed French (or other dark roast) coffee
Grated chocolate, or freshly ground nutmeg (optional)

In a small saucepan combine the milk, chocolate syrup, and almond extract until blended. Bring just to a boil over medium-low heat.

Pour the milk mixture and coffee simultaneously into a French café au lait bowl, or large coffee cup. Top with grated chocolate or freshly ground nutmeg, if desired. Serve immediately. Makes 1 serving.

(*Courtesy:* Coffee Science Organization.)

A CUP FULL OF PERKS

✓ The coffee tree is technically a shrub or plant, but the term "coffee trees" is noted on an estate or plantation.

✓ A versatile beverage—good and bad—continues to get mixed reviews from the scientific world.

✓ Arabica beans are more popular than robusta beans (not as high quality, but they contain more caffeine and are used in coffee blends and instant coffee).

✓ The seed to cup process is a lengthy ordeal from planting, harvesting, processing, exporting, roasting, tasting, and brewing to when the bean is in your cup of java.

✓ Like chocolate, coffee is graded for its quality.

✓ There are four basic coffee roasts—light, medium, medium dark, and dark—and it's the dark roast that boasts the most antioxidant power.

✓ Coffee contains health-boosting antioxidants—the two most important ones are chlorogenic acid and caffeic acid—but there are hundreds of compounds that make coffee a new superfood.

Research, especially in the past decade, shows that quality coffees, both regular and decaf, which are derived from a plant that produces the beans for coffee around the globe, may help you to: lower your risk of heart disease; stave off diabetes; lower the risk of developing cancer; prevent Parkinson's and Alzheimer's disease; slow the aging process; and add years to your life.

In this book, I will show you how using coffee (teamed with other superfoods) no longer deserves a bad rap. But note, it is a wide Coffee World, and knowing which type, how much, when, and why to indulge in the magical beans is key to reaping the benefits of one of the healthiest foods in the world.

You can also get your daily brew from cooking and baking with coffee. I've included dozens of recipes to wake up your palate *and* to help nourish your body, mind, and spirit. And coffee infused in candy, ice cream, cosmetics, candles, and beauty products—and its household uses—will enlighten you, too, with its versatile virtues.

So, pour another cup of coffee—and read on. It's time to get a real taste of the magical beans. Take a fresh look at your everyday coffee lover's findings, from yesteryear and today—and discover exactly why and how this high-octane stuff is one of the world's most powerful and delicious medicines.

An Awakening of Java

Coffee is the common man's gold, and like gold, it brings to every person the feeling of luxury and nobility.

—Sheik Abd-al-Kadir[1]

So while churchgoing had its coffee perks for me as a kid with a restless nature, I now get why monks chewed coffee beans to get through long bouts of prayer. During my grade school years the aroma of coffee awoke me every morning. My parents would rise at 6:00 A.M. five days a week, like the *Groundhog Day* film—repeating the same day as they'd rush to get ready for work and look forward to the 10- to 20-minute coffee break.

In the fifties, America's workplaces were changing and giving workers a break, so to speak. Lunchrooms in office buildings (like my parents worked at) and factories (like my next-door neighbor went to) were part of the work drill. History tells it that The American Coffee Bureau saw a chance to market its coffee and started a campaign with a slogan: "Give Yourself a Coffee Break—Get What Coffee Gives You." And this spawned the coffee break, giving hardworking Americans time out to recharge during the daily grind.[2]

One Monday morning, warm and cozy in bed during a winter storm, I faked sick and took a coffee break day. When I was home alone, I made a coffee concoction from the leftover brew in the coffee percolator on the kitchen countertop. I poured a large copper mug full of java spiked with whole milk and table sugar. I watched Julia Child on *The French Chef*, and coffee commercials—a husband unhappy with his wife's coffee greeted me.

I was happy in my own self-made Coffee World. On the charcoal-colored walls in our family room, I enjoyed the framed posters of places where coffee plants grow: Africa and Costa Rica. Like a coffee plant blossoming with its fragrant flowers, I escaped into my own exotic world. It may not have been in the "bean belt," the area between the Tropics of Cancer and Capricorn, but it was a comfort zone for me, a kid enjoying the novelty of coffee.

While there are no references to the genesis of coffee in the Bible, coffee legend tells the discovery of the first coffee trees in Ethiopia. Coffee originated in a land where wild coffee tree forests are still the primary source of harvested coffee. The coffee tree wasn't given praise like the olive branch or gift of honey in the Old Testament, but the story of the mystical bean with remarkable powers does get noticed by dozens of cultures way, way back in time. . . .

FRISKY GOATS JUST WANNA HAVE FUN

Back in the days of the ancient past, the roots of the coffee plant were accidentally discovered, and it's no surprise that its benefits opened up the eyes of four-leggers and two-leggers. In the Ethiopian highlands, where the legend of Kaldi, the goatherd, originated, coffee trees grow today and they have for centuries. Though we will never know with certainty, there probably is some truth to the Kaldi tale. Legend has it that after eating berries from a certain tree, Kaldi's goats became so spirited that they didn't sleep at night. Kaldi reported his observation to the abbot at the local monastery, who made a drink with the berries and discovered that it kept him alert like the frisky goats for long hours of evening prayer. Soon the abbot had shared his discovery with the other monks at the monastery, and knowledge of the energizing effects of the berries began to spread through the grapevine. . . .

ARABS WAKE UP TO COFFEE

People shared the news about the energizing berries and coffee made its debut on the Arabian Peninsula, triggering excitement like a real-life *E.T.* landing on Earth. Coffee's merits and reputation began to flourish. The Arabs, however, were the first not only to cultivate coffee but also to start its trade. By the fifteenth century, coffee was being grown in the Yemen district of Arabia. Then, by the sixteenth century, the magic of the coffee bean grew noteworthy in Persia, Egypt, Syria, and Turkey.

Its buzz was due, in part, to the Muslims, forbidden alcoholic drinks by the Koran, finding coffee an energizing substitute—and a healthier beverage that enhanced mental and physical efforts. But it doesn't stop there.

HERE COMES COFFEE

European travelers to the Near East joined in the hoopla about the magical coffee beans and brought back stories to share of the must-have dark black beverage. By the 17th century, coffee made its mark in Europe and was getting noticed country by country across the continent. But the unusual beverage didn't go without creating a ruckus.

Despite the uproar about the "evil" beverage in cities of England, Austria, France, Germany, and Holland, coffeehouses were considered good and became hot spots for socializing. In England "penny universities" sprang up for the simple reason that for the price of a penny one could buy a cup of java and chat—healthful to both the mind and body. More than 300 coffeehouses in London attracted people from all walks of life, including merchants, shippers, brokers, and artists.

In the mid-1600s, coffee continued to be the rave and made the cut in New Amsterdam, a location later called New York by the British. Interestingly, coffee upstaged tea, the old drink of choice. Blame it on money matters or politics.

TEA PARTY DUMPS TEA, DRINKS COFFEE

Leading up to the American Revolution, in December 1773 the "Boston Tea Party" was the historical event that began the shift in

America to a coffee-drinking nation—and made a mega statement. Tea was a more popular beverage, but the heavy tax on tea imposed on the American colonies by the British forced the adoption and ultimate national popularity of coffee as the number-one-consumed beverage in America.[3]

COFFEE PLANTATIONS SPROUT . . .

So, as the benefits of coffee added up, from its physical, mental, and monetary virtues, demand soared. Competition to cultivate coffee outside of Arabia was happening. As history has it, Arabs tried to hold on to their moneymaker, but the Dutch succeeded in sharing the good of coffee goods later in the 17th century. India plants failed, but efforts on the island of Java—now Indonesia—succeeded. The coffee berries eaten by goats ended up in widespread cultivation of coffee trees in Sumatra and Celebes.

Big Gifts for Coffee Shakers and Movers

As the story goes, in 1714, the mayor of Amsterdam presented a gift of a young coffee plant to a king, Louis XIV of France, to be planted in the Royal Botanical Garden in Paris. Several years later, a naval officer, Gabriel de Clieu, obtained a seedling from the king's plant. Despite bad weather and pirates during a challenging voyage, he transported it to Martinique. Once it was planted, 18 million coffee trees on the island of Martinique was the result in the next 50 years. It was also the stock from which coffee trees throughout the Caribbean and South and Central America originated. Coffee is believed to have arrived in Brazil in the hands of Francisco de Mello Palheta, who was sent to French Guiana for the purpose of obtaining coffee seedlings. But the French were not willing to share— Palheta did not succeed. Alas, the French governor's wife was charmed by the man, so she offered him a going-away gift of flowers. Buried inside he found enough coffee seeds to begin what is today a billion-dollar industry.[4]

. . . AND COFFEE TREES ABOUND

Coffee, a drink that people in dozens of countries and on seven continents enjoy, ended up with a happy ever after ending as a prized commodity crop. Missionaries, travelers, traders, and colonists saw to it that coffee seeds were transported during travels from place to place and coffee trees were planted around the world.

Coffee plantations and estates began to thrive in tropical forests and on rugged mountain highlands. New nations grew and flourished thanks to coffee trees and their fruit, which produced cherished coffee. By the 19th century coffee made its way to America as a treasured coffee bean and had grown into the world's prized export crop—coffee.

(Courtesy: The National Coffee Association of U.S.A., Inc. [adaptation]).

A BLAST FROM THE PAST—COFFEE CULTURE

Welcome to the coffeehouse or coffee shop of yesteryear, going back centuries ago. Coffeehouses were a place where people would go to savor coffee and for social interaction. The consensus among historians is that the first coffeehouse opened its doors in Constantinople. But there is a disagreement on which one was the first one. It's been said the first café was named Kiva Han, making its debut in 1475. We do know that coffee culture and the coffeehouse go hand in hand.[5]

As time passed, the bloom of coffeehouses spread throughout Western Europe, and Venice—a trade center—in 1615. But coffee, like coffeehouses, did create chaos. Remember the world of Italian Christian leaders who believed the drink was "evil." Despite the uproar, Europe's first coffeehouses began to open their doors, and that spawned the trend.[6]

Not only were coffeehouses—places to drink coffee—blossoming in Europe; they also were teamed with a purpose: business meetings and politics. Banning women was commonplace in England and France. By the mid-1700s, coffeehouses in London were open to a wide clientele—a refuge for the working classes, a social place to go for rest and relaxation. In America, the first popular coffeehouse opened up their doors as early as the 1680s, and the *Mayflower* is said to have used among its cargo a mortar and pestle for grinding its coffee beans.

Teaming cafés with coffee created places where meeting of the minds happened. People of all types gathered at coffeehouses to discuss business, politics, religion, and art. Social interaction at coffeehouses allowed connections among the human race. Surrounding yourself with friends, family, and organizational members can be key to better health and a longer life. Here is a timeline of the names of historical coffeehouses, in chronological order, as coffeehouse history tells it:

- Lloyds of London: History tells it that three Englishmen traveled to Arabia and wrote a report on their findings about coffee. The citizens wanted to try the beverage for themselves and form their own opinion. Impressed, the country's first coffeehouse opened in Oxford in 1650. Two years later, London had its first coffeehouse, too, and more followed. This coffeehouse was the place of businesspeople. Once the end of eighteenth century hit, the coffee drinkers with business on the brain transformed into a company and made the move to their own practice. Before the 1700s, more than 300 coffeehouses were enjoyed in England.[7]
- Penny universities: In the mid-1700s, coffeehouses in Great Britain were called penny universities, probably because one cup of coffee cost one penny. The cost was worth the price to pay because the reward was connecting with people, from scholars to neighbors—at a place where communities, laws, and social attitudes were created.[8]
- The Green Dragon: In 1773, another important coffeehouse in history, The Green Dragon, was the spot where Americans gathered and discussed England's tea tax—and the Continental Congress made coffee the new national beverage.[9]
- Café Foy: Later, in 1789, the French Revolution started at this café, where social activist Camille Desmoulins initiated a revolt.[10]
- The Merchant's Coffeehouse and Tontine Coffeehouse: In 1817, this coffeehouse duo was the place business happened. These two historical coffeehouses morphed into the New York Stock and Exchange Board—and now are known as the New York Stock Exchange.[11]

OTHER PAST MEDICAL USES OF COFFEE

These healing powers discovered by using coffee are noted by numerous coffee historians, past and present-day.

Historical User	Method	Ailment or Benefit
Ethiopians	Coffee	To treat medical conditions; prevent sickness such as the flu[12]
Sheik Gemaleddin, holy man of Aden	Coffee	Improved health[13]
Unknown physician	Coffee	Wrote prescriptions to help sick patients[14]
Arabs from Arabia	Coffee	Enjoyed caffeine benefits[15]
African tribes	Coffee berries mixed with fat	Energizing[16]
German physician Leonhard Rauwolf	Coffee	His book *Rauwolf's Travels* mentioned coffee's health benefits
Europeans	Coffee	A drink to heal illness, such as digestive woes

COFFEE MILESTONES

Year	What Happened	What It Did
10th Century	First mentions of coffee drinking are found in Arab medicinal texts	Proved coffee was consumed for medicinal/religious purposes[17]
1600s	Coffee replaced beer	Coffee was New York's favorite breakfast drink[18]
1600s	An organization called Women's Petition Against Coffee complained that their men were always at the coffeehouses during domestic crisis	Showed that coffee is social comfort[19]
1600s–1700s	London and America enjoyed coffee for its caffeine	Used for its energizing benefits[20]
1880	The Coffee Break is started by working women in Stroughton, Wisconsin, who took morning and afternoon breaks to go home and tend to their chores and grab a cup of coffee from an ever-present pot on the stove	Coffee was a mother's helper during a hard day's work for women in the 19th century[21]
1903	Decaffeinated coffee was invented	Decaf coffee provides an alternative to regular coffee plus benefits—physical and mental[22]
1942	During World War II, American soldiers are issued instant coffee in ration kits	Coffee provides energy, alertness, and a sense of well-being[23]

COFFEE MILESTONES (cont.)

Year	What Happened	What It Did
1951	*Time* magazine notes that since the war the coffee break has been written into union contracts	The coffee break provides time for workers to rest, relax, and socialize for better health[24]
2001	According to a national survey, respondents would give up chocolate and Internet access before giving up coffee	Coffee is a must-have beverage in the 21st century[25]

Discovering the beginnings of the coffee plant country by country makes me, and perhaps you, too, respect each cup of coffee savored. While I appreciate all types of roasts and flavored coffees, iced coffee drinks are a treat, especially if they are of an exotic nature. The following recipe is cold, sweet, and boasts a touch of pizzazz with its classic Coca-Cola—a drink of choice I drank straight from the bottle as a teenager. If you're calorie-counting or don't want the extra sugar, turn to diet cola. Enjoy the taste of Brazil—a country where coffee is sacred and historical.

Brazilian Iced Chocolate

❖ ❖ ❖

2 ounces unsweetened chocolate
1¾ ounces sugar
8 fluid ounces double-strength coffee

20 fluid ounces milk
12 fluid ounces Coca-Cola
Whipped cream or ice cream
Ice cubes

Melt chocolate in bain-marie over hot water. Stir in sugar. Gradually stir in hot coffee, mixing thoroughly. Add milk and continue cooking until all particles of chocolate are dissolved and mixture is smooth—about 10 minutes. Pour into jar, cover, and chill. When ready to serve, stir in chilled Coca-Cola. Serve over ice cubes in tall glasses. Top with either whipped or ice cream. Makes 5 cups.

(*Courtesy:* The Roast and Post Coffee Company; www. realcoffee.co.uk.)

I brewed this coffee recipe as is—except I did turn to Diet Coke. It's a different coffee treat—and yes, there is a caffeine buzz from the cola, coffee, and sugar. The Brazilian coffee beverage was a treat on a hot, dry summer afternoon at Lake Tahoe and I didn't have to book a flight to South America to enjoy the refreshing java juice. Topping the cream with a dash of cinnamon or chocolate shavings gives it an extra taste and presentation that'll wow both chocolate and coffee lovers.

Coffee's energizing powers from legendary times throughout the centuries was touted to have health attributes. Despite the thumbs-down it has received in the 20th century from doctors and nutritionists claiming its downside, from caffeine to empty calories when spoiled with sugar and cream, it's made a splash in research worldwide in the 21st century.

These days coffee is getting kudos from scientists, medical doctors, nutritionists, and this is making coffee lovers, like me, smile. In the next chapter, "A Historical Testimony," I'll show you exactly how coffee is getting the respect it's earned and deserves and why we should be appreciative to dancing goats in the night and their observant caretaker.

A CUP FULL OF PERKS

✓ Coffee was discovered in Ethiopia by a goatherd and his dancing goats and noted for its energizing benefits for man.

✓ Coffee made its name in Arabia and other countries on into Europe. It was used for its amazing powers and was exported to London, where coffeehouses, places where people gathered to drink coffee and socialize for business and pleasure, began.

✓ In the 18th century the Boston Tea Party was a revolt against the tax on tea and Americans turned to coffee as the beverage of choice.

✓ Budget-smart coffee was brought by man to America and was touted for its usefulness for mind, body, and spirit.

✓ Coffee roasters and retailers as well as advocates of the healing powers of coffee paved the path of its usefulness and demand in the 1900s.

✓ By the mid-20th century and into the 21st century, coffee roasters and retailers had developed a reputation as providing a beverage that was here to stay in America and around the world.

PART 2

COFFEE:
THE
MAGICAL BEANS

A Historical Testimony

*The coffee was boiling over a charcoal fire, and
large slices of bread and butter were piled one upon
the other like deals in a lumber yard.*
—Charles Dickens (1812–1870)[1]

Coffee in different forms treated my preteen, green taste buds. My budding imagination took me to foreign lands where coffee trees grow and flourish and people enjoy sophisticated coffee drinks. I observed adults sipping coffee spiked with alcohol and non-alcohol. It was intriguing to discover a new spin on the beverage that was forbidden for kids like me to drink.

After one dinner party at our home, my mother (coffee must have been the gift that gave her boundless energy) served slices of cheesecake paired with a dark-colored coffee in small white porcelain cups. I asked her, "What is this dark stuff?" She answered, "Espresso. I drank it in a bistro in Paris." Since her trip to Europe, when I was in the third grade, she came back home with coffee attitude.

Served in a 3-ounce demitasse (espresso cups) the beverage presentation looked cute, like something in an *Alice in Wonderland* scene. I wanted to taste the strange, dark brew but was timid. It looked like the coffee cup picture on the cover of a French menu that my mom brought home from her trip abroad to France, Spain, and Italy. Actually, the Italian-sounding "espresso" word (which I incorrectly pronounced "expresso") originated in France in the late 1800s and was appreciated in Italy later.

So, I shut my eyes (like diving off a block into a cold pool at swim club) and sipped the dark mud. "This tastes awful!" I exclaimed. I was still a kid (like a coffee plant that had not fully matured); what did I know? I swapped my coffee for a bowl of coffee ice cream with chocolate syrup.

At the same time, during the 20th century, coffee roasters and retailers were also discovering what titillated the palates of Americans. Coffee company pioneers understood the demand for the caffeinated brew, from workplaces with coffee breaks to coffeehouses. They knew that coffee had a place both at work and play. And these findings have been embraced and are now expanding to buzz-worthy health news effects of coffee for the mainstream audience.

COFFEE GIANTS IN THE TWENTIETH CENTURY

Some of the noteworthy coffee producers of the world made history in the 20th century and paved the way for the 21st-century coffee companies on the West Coast of America and worldwide. Also, what is so interesting is that many of these groundbreaking pioneers are family generation run and have ties back to the 1900s. By the mid-20th century, coffee was a staple beverage in the average American home and on the road. The popularity of cars and highways made traveling more common, and stopping at a coffee shop or diner for coffee and a bite to eat was a trend that became a mainstay. When I was a kid growing up in the fifties, my parents ordered coffee at coffee shops before our lunch or dinner made its way to the table. And after the meal coffee was served, too.

WAKING UP TO MAJOR COFFEE BRANDS

When I began my exploration to discover who's who in coffee companies, I quickly learned that there wasn't an updated, tidy, ready-made list compiled of well-known top coffee brands. I discovered that, as with some chocolate moguls, some mergers of big-name coffee companies have made big changes in the past years.

Indeed, major coffee corporations still fuel the supply of large institutions such as hospitals, office buildings, and universities as well as households: Philip Morris/Altria Group (Kraft and Maxwell House), J.M. Smucker Company (Folgers, Millstone), and MZB-USA (Hills Bros., MJB and Chase and Sanborn).[2]

Here's the lowdown, at a glance in chronological time sequence, of the major coffee giants—from past to present as the major coffee companies continue to keep coffee lovers smiling.

Folgers: Welcome to an established company founded back in 1850 in San Francisco, near my home. It has been touted as an iconic American brand that has made great-tasting coffee for more than 150 years. In the 21st century, The Folgers Coffee Company merged with the J.M. Smucker Company. Folgers is keeping up with the whirlwind of coffee trends and offers instant to gourmet, whole bean to ground, mild to dark-roasted blends as well as decaf and flavored coffee.[3]

Eight o'Clock: Like Folgers, this coffee brand has also enjoyed the limelight for more than a century and a half, with the first store beginning back in 1859. This company stays on top of their game by keeping up with the demand and offering a blend of 100 percent arabica coffee, original, decaf, 100 percent Colombian, 50 percent decaf, and flavored coffees.[4]

Maxwell House: Staying in line with the major players, another super coffee brand, Maxwell House—today a household name—was first created in 1892 at a Nashville, Tennessee, hotel, the Maxwell House Hotel. Legend has it in 1907 a cup of Maxwell House coffee was served to President Theodore Roosevelt and he was overheard to comment that it was "good to the last drop."

Later, the Cheek-Neal Coffee Company registered the trademark slogan "Maxwell House Good to the last drop" in 1926. The Postum Cereal Company purchased the assets of Cheek-Neal, including Maxwell House Coffee, in 1928, and, through several corporate acquisitions, became General Goods in 1929. In 1989, Kraft and General Foods combined to form Kraft General Foods, which owns Maxwell House Coffee today.[5]

Yuban: This major coffee company gets deserved attention. At the turn of the century, a young coffee merchant named John Arbuckle was on the quest for the perfect cup of coffee for his Yuletide Banquet. A small shipment of coffee from South America caught his eye—later earning the title Yu-Ban. This brand, part of Kraft Foods, promotes itself as being green by helping protect the environment and supporting the people and wildlife in coffee-growing regions.[6]

Chock full o'Nuts: In the 20th century before I was born, this brand started in a New York store, in 1932, and is the sixth largest coffee brand. After the depression struck, even William Black's nuts seemed too much of a luxury. So he converted his chain of 18 nut shops into small coffee shops, selling a good cup of coffee and a sandwich for a nickel. In 1953 William Black began to sell his own brand of coffee in grocery stores and decided to name it after his original street-side nut shop—Chock full o'Nuts. In December 2005, Chock full o'Nuts was purchased by Massimo Zanetti Beverages, USA. With over 30 different beverages to choose from, they offer something for everyone.[7]

Starbucks: Starbucks history starts back in 1971 when the first store opened in Seattle, Washington. The store initially sold just coffee beans and coffee-making equipment rather than the drinks they have become famous for. Over the course of its life Starbucks has bought or acquired companies such as Peet's and Seattle's Best Coffee. Today Starbucks has expanded to more than 17,000 stores in 55 countries around the world. Their biggest presence is still in the United States, with 11,000 locations. You can find a Starbucks in such diverse nations as Chile, Romania, Bahrain, Bulgaria, and Budapest.[8]

Millstone: After Starbucks made a splash in the coffee world, it didn't stop other coffee companies in Washington from opening their doors. For Millstone, it began in 1981 when Phil Johnson started selling 5-pound sacks of whole-bean arabicas to gourmet shops in the Seattle area. This marked the start of supplying supermarkets fresh, high-quality whole-bean bulk coffee.[9]

A Grounded Coffee Company with Roots

MZB-USA: As the story goes, Mr. Massimo Zanetti's grandfather sold coffee. So did his father. So does he. The difference is that his grandfather and father were in the business of green coffee. Mr. Massimo Zanetti was the first in the family to produce and sell roasted coffee. That was 35 years ago, and at that time the company was selling about a ton of roasted coffee a year.

Today, the company, with the parent company based in Bologna, Italy, offers a wide range of premium coffee and sells 120,000 tons of coffee annually and processes 2.5 million bags of green coffee per year. Its operations include a coffee plantation and green coffee processing plant in Brazil, a coffee mill in Costa Rica, a green coffee export company in these two markets, and a green coffee trading company in Switzerland.

It runs nine roasting plants around the world and boasts a worldwide distribution network of subsidiaries and authorized dealers in 100 countries, production of professional espresso machines and bar equipment under the La San Marco name, and a network of over 700 international coffee shops.

Some of the brands being handled by MZB include Chock full o'Nuts, Hills Bros., Hills Bros. Cappuccino, Segafredo Zanetti, Chase and Sanborn, MJB, Corporate Brands and Segafredo Cafes, and Kauai Coffee from the Garden Island. These days, MZB-USA is keeping up with health-conscious consumers by offering a wide selection of coffees, including decaf, half caffeinated, premium coffees, and flavored coffees.[10]

5 QUESTIONS FOR
JOE A. VINSON—
"COFFEE IS OUR NUMBER ONE SOURCE
OF ANTIOXIDANTS"

While coffee company players make the news, researchers, such as Joe A. Vinson, Ph.D., from the University of Scranton in Pennsylvania, made a big buzz about the world's favorite beverage, too. In 2005, he discovered that the average American consumes most of his antioxidants (healthy compounds) from coffee. Vinson and his research team analyzed over 100 foods and beverages and then compared the intake of these foods to that of the diet in the United States. The results were surprising and the professor made his mark showing that coffee is a top-ranking winner in the world of disease-fighting antioxidant foods and beverages. While his past research has gone down in history, he continues to study superfoods. Recently, I asked him some follow-up questions right before his new research that shows red potatoes are rich in antioxidants, too.

Q: Back in 2005, you said: "Most people drink it for the caffeine." You added, "But it's the number one source of antioxidants in the U.S. diet." Is this fact true?
A: Yes.

Q: Does decaf have antioxidants?
A: Decaf has 20 percent less polyphenols than caffeinated coffee, but this is not significantly lower.

Q: Are there hundreds of antioxidant compounds found in coffee? Why is the mix important and not just chlorogenic acid and caffeic acid?
A: There are hundreds of compounds and the effects of pure compounds are never as large as a combination of compounds.

Q: You found the average person gets 1,299 milligrams of antioxidants daily from coffee. The closest competition was teas at 294 milligrams.
A: Coffee contribution is revised to 691 milligrams/day and total from all foods and beverages is revised to 2056 mg/day of polyphenols.

Q: Does the French Paradox come into play with coffee?
A: The French consume 30 percent more per capita than does the U.S.A. So coffee is an essential part of the French lifestyle, the Mediterranean Diet.

COOL COFFEEHOUSES IN THE 20TH CENTURY . . .

Speaking of the French Mediterranean, the 20th-century coffeehouses actually rooted from the popular espresso bars in Italian-American communities, such as Greenwich Village and San Francisco's North Beach. These coffee shops glorified coffee in the Bohemian Beatnik era of the 1950s—the decade I was born in and grew up to experience the coffeehouse phenomenon.

In the 1960s it was a time when poets and folk singers, from Bob

Dylan to Joan Baez, paved the way to a cool hangout where antiestablishment young people sipped black coffee, smoked cigarettes, talked politics, and socialized. In my teens, I recall hitchhiking in the sixties north to San Francisco, where coffeehouses were a place to meet strangers and escape.

Once Starbucks made its mark in the coffee world in the early seventies, coffee shops became an American trend that swept through the nation on into the 21st century and offered an array of coffee specialty drinks to coffee lovers.

In the late 20th century, coffeehouses became more sophisticated in their coffee selection, and today they are places where you can order coffee roasts from around the world, flavored coffees, organic coffee, and hot and cold coffee drinks and have an espresso bar type of atmosphere. Bookstores, including Barnes & Noble, offer coffee and snacks, from bagels to cookies. These are places where people set up their laptops to work or play, as well as interact with others.

Socializing contributed to the rise of coffeehouses. Like centuries ago, people sit and enjoy coffee, which provides not only health aspects in relaxing and communicating but also a dose of healthful coffee, which was and still is part of the coffeehouse package that is here to stay. As time passed, in the 1980s and 1990s coffee shops and family-style restaurants served regular coffee, meals, and pies. As a kid who lived through the coffeehouse period, I experienced the transformation—and I worked as a waitress serving coffee to people (all ages).

These days, in the 21st century, during financial ups and downs, coffee is still a beverage that people enjoy at coffee shops that specialize in coffee, like the giant coffee chains Starbucks and Peet's. It's the caffeine jolt to the flavor of specialty coffee drinks made by a barista that keeps the coffee shop in America alive. These places that offer java in all sizes, shapes, and flavors are places where people go to relax and work. Even though I've never been to a European café, I have been to European-style bistros in San Francisco and on the Bay Area peninsula up to Lake Tahoe. Cafés with a European flair offer an outdoor terrace or sidewalk with seats, tables, and umbrellas. Once a place for solely face-to-face socialization, in the nineties, cafés in America were becoming hot spots to use computers. Computers and Internet access in a café or bookstore with an espresso bar that offers Wi-Fi—a place to work and relax. And coffee shops, like these, continue to be a mainstay in the United States as well as around the world.

... TO 21ST-CENTURY CAFÉ CULTURE

Coffeehouses are a mainstay in different countries and coffee is different among the variety of cultures. So, if you travel to one of these regions and are in search of a coffee fix, this is what you might find; so say tourists to locals and coffee roasters to historians, who've been there, done that coffee thing in these regions:

Arab World/Turkey Coffeehouses. In the Arab World coffeehouses serve coffee (*qahwa/kahwa*) and tea. In these places dominated by men and boys, beverages are enjoyed while playing chess, watching television, and smoking shisha.

Australia Cafés. Coffee shops down under have been popular with the Aussies since the fifties. Roasted specialty coffee and "Flat-White," a coffee drink, are popular these days, especially in Melbourne, a spot for students and artists.

China Coffeehouse Chains. Drinking coffee (*kafei*) is a pastime for businesspeople who are on the go. The price of coffee in China is said to be higher than in the United States, but it's worth the price because of the image that goes with frequenting coffeehouse chains.

French Cafés. Welcome to a brasserie that serves coffee (*café*), meals, and single dishes and is more casual than French restaurants. A bistro is a combo café/restaurant in Paris. Coffee spots like these are for intellectuals.

Malaysia and Singapore Coffee Shops. Asian coffee shops are a bit more traditional than others I've discussed. That said, you can expect to get coffee (*kopi*) and breakfast, including eggs and toast.

Middle East Coffeehouses. Here are gathering spots for men, like the Arab-Turkey spots, to drink Arabic coffee (*mashboot*) or tea, listen to music, read books, and play chess and backgammon.

Netherlands Coffee Shops. If the Middle East coffeehouses surprise you, drinking coffee (*kaffee*) in the Netherlands, like in Denmark, may shock you, too: They offer beverages and legalized marijuana.

Norway Coffee Shops. These are places to meet and grab a cup of *kaffee* while en route to and from work.

United Kingdom Coffee Chains. Coffee drinking in the UK is often found at chains like Starbucks and Coffee Republic, and it's the young professionals who gravitate to these places.

OTHER 20TH-TO-21ST-CENTURY HEALTH MILESTONES

Coffee continued to raise eyebrows in the 1900s as it swept the nation and world with its feel-good compounds and social benefits. And, its healing powers are becoming more buzzworthy in the 21st century.

Year	What Happened	Author/Doctor/Company
1901	Instant coffee made its debut	Attributed to a Japanese-American chemist, Saton Kato
1939	Coffee was consumed for its stimulating effect	White-Kobrick Coffee Company was formed
1940s	The popular phrase "cup of joe" referring to a cup of coffee	U.S. Army used the term; popularized by enlisted men during WWII
1971	Seattle, Washington, a place where Starbucks and coffee-houses became an American trend	Founders: Jerry Baldwin, Zev Siegl, Alfred Peet; Howard Schultz is CEO
2005	Groundbreaking research on antioxidants in coffee	Joe Vinson, Ph.D.
2011	Studies on compounds in coffee and how they help lower the risk of developing diseases	Scientists worldwide

(*Courtesy:* Gourmet-Coffee-Zone.com)

COFFEE IS TIMELESS

Past and present, coffee is a food that stimulates the minds of entrepreneurs and creative artisans in America and around the world. Coffee and its health benefits were making the news in the late 20th century and continue to do so in the 21st century.

And it's not uncommon to find people in the Coffee World, from roasters and retailers to coffee lovers, simple and sophisticated, to savor the magical beans and the good that they can do for the body and mind.

Coffee beverages complete with flavorings and spices can wow coffee people—and these drinks (alcoholic and non-alcoholic) have a long history from different countries, including Europe, in past centuries. Coffee desserts are often paired with coffees—regular roasts and specialty drinks—like this timeless recipe created by a seasoned cook with Italian roots:

Cappuccino Crème Brûlée

❖ ❖ ❖

4 eggs, beaten
1 (12-ounce) can low-fat
   evaporated milk
¼ cup sugar (or to taste)
½ teaspoon salt
½ teaspoon nutmeg and/
   or cinnamon
1 tablespoon Marsala
   Olive Oil

1 teaspoon vanilla
½ teaspoon Danish pastry
   extract (Watkins)
1 tablespoon instant
   espresso coffee powder
1 teaspoon cocoa
¼ cup sugar to sprinkle tops
   (turbinado)

Preheat oven to 325°F. Lightly grease eight 4-ounce custard cups. Combine eggs, milk, sugar, salt, nutmeg, olive oil, and flavorings in mixing bowl. Pour mixture into custard cups evenly. Place cups in deep baking pan; add enough water to pan to come halfway up sides of cups. Cover loosely with foil. Bake 30 to 35 minutes or until cake tester comes out clean from center. Let cool in pan; remove; place on wire rack to cool completely.

> To serve, sprinkle evenly with sugar, and place under broiler until caramelized, watching closely as not to burn, about 1 minute. The caramelized topping becomes brittle, creating a delicious flavor and texture contrast to the smooth, creamy custard beneath. Serves 6 to 8.
>
> (*Courtesy:* Gemma Sanita Sciabica, *Baking Sensational Sweets with California Olive Oil.*)

Now that I've put coffee on the time table, it's time to analyze its healthful ingredients like a mysterious wonder (mesmerizing scientists). Yes, it's time to take a close-up and personal view of what components make coffee a superfood, amazing researchers time after time. I tackle this controversial nutrition topic in the next chapter.

A CUP FULL OF PERKS

✓ The United States is a hot spot for coffee retailers and importers, but it's the coffee belt countries where the superfood is grown and nurtured, to be exported around the world.
✓ Old-time coffee corporations, aka the giants, include Kraft and Maxwell House, Procter & Gamble, and Nestlé, which supply major outlets, from universities to hospitals.
✓ Other well-known coffee companies have made their name in both the 20th and 21st centuries. These major players include: Chock full o'Nuts, Eight o'Clock, Millstone, and Yuban.
✓ The West Coast's coffee retailers, including Peet's and Starbucks, are touted for their coffee products and coffee shops.
✓ While coffee companies are busy working in the coffee industry, medical researchers, such as Dr. Joe Vinson, are aware of the growing trend of the healing powers of coffee.
✓ The coffee industry in the 21st century has captured a worldwide audience and coffee shops are still a popular trend for their coffee and as places for socializing.

Where Are the Secret Ingredients?

*Without my morning coffee I'm just like a dried up
piece of roast goat.*
—Johann Sebastian Bach (1685–1750), "The Coffee
  Cantata"[1]

As a curious teenager, I began to branch out with my coffee astuteness like a coffee plant in bloom. I noticed how coffee—a beverage that can have a stimulating effect on humans due to its caffeine content—played a role in my friends' households. It had its stimulating effects but also its comforting wholesomeness. Coffee wasn't just a beverage for a morning jolt to go to work—it had a multitude of uses and I was beginning to witness its versatile nature.

One Sunday afternoon I visited my best pal, Deb, who lived in the corner yellow house with a white picket fence. In the den, her extended family drank coffee spiked with table sugar. The smell from cigarettes and a hectic pace while her mother and father did other things, instead of enjoying coffee drinking (like in the Middle East, South America, and Asia), made me feel uneasy. I fled on my skateboard to my other friend's home down the street—a down-to-earth oasis and the home of a person who knew how to enjoy her coffee amid Mother Nature.

I found Lois in her backyard amid a garden of tomato vines, blackberry bushes, orange and lemon trees. My earthy pal was in a comfortable pose, sitting on a wooden bench, sipping black coffee from a large ceramic coffee mug. She untangled her long, straight wet locks in the sun while munching on a toasted slice of homemade bread spread with fruit jam that her mother had canned. Their cat basked in the sunshine; her dog ran free amid the backyard. The fresh aroma of the steaming hot fresh brew that she poured from a thermos and the mood of calm amid nature's finest mesmerized me.

These days, in the 21st century, folks like my old-time friends are reaping the same caffeine jolt and creature comforts of coffee—but we now know the beverage has more to it and is healthful no matter why you drink it.

One ounce of coffee, for instance, brewed from grounds, prepared with tap water, contains zero calories, cholesterol, and fat. It has almost 12 milligrams of caffeine, trace elements of saturated fat, magnesium, phosphorus, and protein.[2]

When you look at coffee's ingredients per one ounce (which doesn't appear on coffee bags) it appears to be an empty nutritional beverage, right? But 8 ounces in your basic brewed cup of java without additives is a different story that'll wake you up to coffee's new status as a superfood.

More Coffee, Please

Although coffee is 99 percent water, the coffee beans provide your diet with small quantities of other vitamins and minerals. An 8-ounce cup of coffee contains all of the following (caffeine will vary depending on the quality and brand of coffee):

Nutrient	Quantity	% Daily Value
Riboflavin	.18 mg	10.59%
Pantothenic Acid	.602 mg	6.02%
Zinc	5 mg	3.33%
Potassium	116 mg	3.31%

Manganese	.055 mg	2.75%
Niacin	.453 mg	2.27%
Thiamin	.033 mg	2.20%
Magnesium	7 mg	1.75%
Folate	5 mg	1.25%
Phosphorus	7 mg	.70%
Protein	.28 mg	.56%
Calcium	5 mg	.50%
Vitamin K	.2 mg	.25%
Sodium	5 mg	.21%
Iron	.02 mg	.11%
Vitamin E	.02 mg	.10%
Copper	.002 mg	.10%
Vitamin B-6	.001 mg	.05%

(*Courtesy:* USDA National Nutrient Database for Standard Reference, SR18. 8 ounces coffee, brewed from grounds, prepared with tap water, page 20. Used with permission from the Oldways Conference on Refreshingly Good News for Coffee Lovers, New York, NY 2006.)

COFFEE'S CAFFEINE-O-METER

During my trek through Coffee World, the words "coffee is chock-full of caffeine" echoed from one nutritionist to another—and some would lecture about how pairing the liquid jolt with sugar, artificial flavorings, cream, and whipped cream was worse than committing a mortal sin (or I felt that way after our thumbs-down-on-coffee conversations). I sensed that many of these food experts didn't go the distance to learn the dietary value of coffee (in moderation).

The virtues of coffee are plentiful and its caffeine content has its virtues, too. Actually, the caffeine content of coffee varies a lot and for the most part isn't off the charts unless you drink cup after cup—which is not recommended by me or health professionals, from doctors to nutritionists. When looking at my caffeine-o-meter, most folks don't have the real coffee spoon scoop on how much caffeine is in their cup of java.

Here's the word about caffeine at a glance: instant coffee: 65 milligrams; fresh-brewed coffee: 100 to 130 milligrams; espresso: 65 milligrams; decaf: 5 to 30 milligrams. And, of course, the brand, quality, and strength of the coffee beans can affect the amount of caffeine in coffee.

I learned years ago, thanks to a worker at a Starbucks store, that lighter roasts contain more caffeine than darker roasts. Recently, I discovered espresso doesn't have the intense caffeine fix that its reputation makes it out to have. Espresso coffee contains about one-third the caffeine of a brewed cup of coffee, thanks to the smaller serving size, which is less than a normal cup of coffee. Blame it, too, on the fact that espresso comes from premium arabica beans (as noted in chapter 1, arabica beans have less caffeine than the robust beans found in many coffee blends).

So how much caffeine in coffee is too much, anyhow? The rules, outlined by the American Dietetic Association (www.eatright.org), are a personal thing. Caffeine consumption is not mathematical: it's individual. Caffeine sensitivity depends on the amount and frequency of caffeine consumption, body weight, physical condition, and overall anxiety level, among other factors. For most healthy adults, moderate amounts of caffeine—200 to 300 milligrams a day, or about two to three cups of coffee—pose no physical problems. However, there are reasons why you might need to reduce your caffeine consumption, including if you're pregnant or nursing or have a medical problem. If you are looking to cut back on your caffeine consumption, start by doing so gradually; then try these tips:

- Mix half regular with half decaffeinated coffee or tea.
- Drink decaffeinated coffee or tea.

- Keep a cup of water alongside your caffeinated beverage and alternate sips to prevent mindless caffeine drinking.

The American Heart Association, like the ADA, is on the java-in-moderation bandwagon. Whether the high caffeine intake increases the risk of coronary heart disease is still under study. Many studies, they say, have been done to see if there's a direct link between caffeine, coffee drinking, and coronary heart disease. The results are conflicting. This may be due to the way the studies were done and confounding dietary factors. So, moderate coffee drinking (one or two cups per day) doesn't seem to be harmful. Counting caffeine milligrams can be tricky, especially since caffeine can also be found in tea, soda, chocolate, cold medication, and pain relievers. So, check out nutritional labels and be coffee caffeine aware.

HOW MUCH CAFFEINE IS IN YOUR CUP OF JOE?

Coffees	Service Size	Caffeine (mg)
Coffee, generic brewed	8 oz.	133 (range: 102–200) (16 oz. = 266)
Starbucks Brewed Coffee (Grande)	16 oz.	320
Einstein Bros. regular coffee	16 oz.	300
Dunkin' Donuts regular coffee	16 oz.	206
Starbucks Vanilla Latte	16 oz.	150
Coffee, generic instant	8 oz.	93 (range: 27–173)
Starbucks Espresso, doppio	2 oz.	150
Starbucks Frappuccino Blended Coffee Beverages, Average	9.5 oz.	115

Coffees	Service Size	Caffeine (mg)
Starbucks Espresso, solo	1 oz.	75
Einstein Bros. Espresso	1 oz.	75
Espresso, generic	1 oz.	40 (range: 30–90)
Starbucks Espresso decaffeinated	1 oz.	4

(*Courtesy:* Center for Science in the Public Interest.)

My Coffee Fix Made a Wrong Turn

Drinking one 12-ounce cup of fresh-brewed coffee every morning is my normal ritual. Several years ago, it was an 8-ounce cup of instant coffee. Then, one day it happened. I changed my routine. A longtime friend from the San Francisco Bay Area paid me a visit. Okay, it was an ex-boyfriend and that in itself put the pressure on me to clean house, get my hair highlighted, manicure/pedicure, and wash the fur kids.

Once Mr. Ex arrived, it was exciting at first. But as the minutes led into a few hours, tension filled the air. It was the same arguments, the same old stuff that split us up. After a dog-cat spat, we agreed to take a drive around Lake Tahoe. But note, I'm sensitive and I sensed he really didn't want to partake in this activity. So, on the road I decided I wanted to stop at a coffee shop and get a latte to go. Worse, I ordered a large coffee.

Fifteen minutes later, my heart was racing, and I got hit with that telltale awful fight-or-flight syndrome. I wanted to flee from the car, from Mr. Ex, and go home. And I did just that.

Like many people, I survived on too much caffeine, which put me in high anxiety mode. For me the problem was a spooky case of coffee nerves, nothing a couple of cups of chamomile tea and time wouldn't heal. I know now how much my body can handle and I abide by my coffee budget.

COFFEE'S AMAZING ANTIOXIDANT POWER

But the disease-fighting, age-defying antioxidants are the big part of coffee's healing powers. Coffee gurus (researchers who analyze it like it's a strange creature with incredible secrets) will tell you that coffee is not just touted for its caffeine power—which is linked to lowering the risk of developing diseases and ailments. As I mentioned in chapter 1, "The Power of Coffee," coffee is antioxidant rich and that's where the real power perks. We're talking mighty disease-fighting antioxidants—the good guys that help to keep your body healthy and stall Father Time.

Two mighty antioxidants—chlorogenic acids and caffeic acid—are given credit for health benefits. Both are mighty antioxidants, and coffee beans are believed to be one of the richest dietary sources of chlorogenic acid on earth. You may consume as much as 70 percent of the total amount of your dietary intake of these two antioxidants.[3]

Coffee boasts other health-boosting antioxidants, including benzoic acids, cinnamic acids, coumarins, flavonoids, lignans, lignins, proanthocyanidins, and stilbenes. But that's not all. . . .

So, what is the roast that contains the most antioxidants in your cup of coffee—medium or dark? If you think bold, darker coffee is better for you, you may be spot-on; so say scientists at the University of British Columbia, who discovered the coffee roast with more antioxidants is a darker roast, sort of.

Past research reveals that antioxidants in coffee showed that coffee could be linked to caffeine or the chlorogenic acid in green coffee beans. But recent findings point to the Maillard reaction (the roasting process of coffee beans), which may be the source of antioxidants, says Yazheng Liu, the lead author of a new study published in *Food Research International*.[4]

Still, while these British Columbia scientists reported increased antioxidants in coffee made from a dark roast, other researchers found a decrease. Some scientists tout the medium-roast coffee for having the most antioxidants. "We have yet to fully decipher all the complex compounds in roasted coffee beans," admits David D. Kitts, co-author of the study. But there is more. . . .

JAVA JUICE HAS MORE FIBER THAN OJ

Not only does your cup of coffee in the morning contain caffeine and plenty of nutrients; it's got dietary fiber, too. Researchers discovered in a Spanish study, published in the *Journal of Agricultural Food Chemistry*, that "brewed coffee contained a significantly higher amount of soluble dietary fiber . . . than other common beverages."

That means coffee, like fiber-rich oat bran and apples, can help lower total cholesterol and LDL cholesterol (the bad stuff), lessening the risk of developing heart disease, and can also help regulate blood sugar for people with diabetes.[5]

ENHANCED "HEALTHIFIED" COFFEE

Some people believe healing coffee can be made even better with its ready-made antioxidants, caffeine, minerals, and vitamins. Despite its new health food reputation, some companies are enhancing the good stuff and believe they are making it even better.

Organo Gold, for one, makes a line of healthy coffee that is claimed to be a "Healthier Coffee" packed with the goodness of the 100 percent certified Ganoderma Lucida Red Mushrooms. There is question about whether Ganoderma provides health effects. The Federal Drug Administration has not evaluated the product but has not given it a thumbs-down, either.

Just ask Regenia Blackmon how this enhanced coffee works and she'll tell you it works wonders for her. She suffers from less joint pain and says she wakes up without the groggy feeling with which coffee used to leave her once the caffeine wore off. "It gives energy without dehydrating the body," she said. What's more, she likes the flavor: "It's a better tasting smooth kind of coffee without the acidic taste afterward."[6]

While this supercoffee sounds super, I'm already a bit overwhelmed with the different coffees in my kitchen waiting for me to try. So, I gave a sample packet to my sibling, a rat-like human who is an honest critic. The flavors include Gourmet Latte and Gourmet Mocha. His critique was not one to write home about, but we don't always see eye to eye. The packets are still in my pantry. Perhaps I'll wait until our next summer or winter blackout. But I am not tossing them, so it's safe to say I will give these supercoffees a taste. Yet I still am unclear why anyone would want to enhance coffee when it's already got so much antioxidant power—why try to fix it when it's working?

SO, HOW MUCH COFFEE IS . . . TOO MUCH?

Here I sit mulling over coffee in my kitchen and wondering, *How many cups can I enjoy each day?* Well, I made the rounds to book authors, scientists, medical doctors, registered dietitians, and the American Heart Association (AHA).

The exact amount varies, depending on your heart health and tolerance. Some doctors believe if you have any heart problems or anxiety woes, stick to decaf or one cup of coffee per day. If you're pregnant— one cup (and no more than 200 milligrams of caffeine per day)—or no coffee is the recommended dose.

Other coffee gurus do not have a problem drinking three cups of coffee per day—and that was the average amount for Americans back in the 1950s. It went like this: one cup in the morning, one in the afternoon, and espresso with dessert after dinner. If you're concerned about caffeine, try regular or decaf in recipes, like this one with superfoods.

Tortellini with Coffee Creole Cream, Broccoli, and Shrimp

❖ ❖ ❖

9-ounce package fresh cheese-filled tortellini, cooked al dente
1 tablespoon olive oil
6 small green onions (scallions), minced
2 cloves garlic
1 cup broccoli florets
½ lb. medium shrimp, peeled and deveined

2 teaspoons Cajun spice blend
1 tablespoon finely ground coffee, regular or decaffeinated
1 tablespoon tomato paste
1 cup cream (or light cream)
Salt to taste
Optional: ¼ cup freshly grated Parmesan or Romano cheese for garnish

Set aside the cooked tortellini to chill while preparing the recipe. Heat the oil in a large nonstick sauté pan and add the green onions, garlic, and broccoli florets. Sauté over medium heat for 1 minute, adding a sprinkle of water to prevent sticking if needed. Add the shrimp, Cajun spices, coffee, and tomato paste, stirring well to lightly brown. Add the cream and stir in to combine all ingredients well, forming a light pink, creamy sauce. Add the cooked tortellini to the mixture and stir well. Cook for 3 minutes until a smooth sauce is formed around the pasta and shrimp. Season to taste with salt. Makes 2–3 servings.

(*Courtesy:* National Coffee Association of U.S.A., Inc., Coffee Science Source.)

It doesn't take a coffee researcher to tell you that coffee is a superfood with good-for-you nutrients—but it helps. So, the question is: Since coffee does pack a powerful punch of antioxidants, compounds, vitamins, and minerals, how does this ancient essential elixir (called a drug) that is available and legal to us in the modern day help your body inside and outside to prevent disease? Scientists, medical doctors, and folks in the coffee industry dished to me about coffee and its benefits, so I discovered what I wanted to know, and you'll find out more about how coffee heals and about its amazing healing powers in the next chapter.

A Cup Full of Perks

✓ In the 21st century, coffee is touted for its caffeine, antioxidants, vitamins, and minerals.
✓ Coffee is praised for its other health virtues: It has no fat, no cholesterol, and no sodium.
✓ Nutritionists in the United States debate about the pros and cons of the health merits of coffee, for a variety of reasons, including caffeine and high fat or sugary flavoring.
✓ The quality of coffee matters. It's organic, fresh, dark-roasted filtered coffee that is the superfood researchers applaud.
✓ It's premium black coffee—without artificial flavored syrup, table

sugar, cream, or whipped cream—that is what nutritionists recommend for health-minded coffee lovers.

✓ Coffee is advised by researchers for its compounds that may help stave off a wide variety of diseases and ailments. However, as with dark chocolate and pure honey, moderation is key.

Coffee, the New Health Food

*Moderately drunk, coffee removes vapours from the
brain, occasioned by fumes of wine, or other strong
liquors; eases pains in the head, prevents sour belch-
ings, and provokes appetite.*
—"England's Happiness Improved" (1699)[1]

In the late sixties, as I was growing up like a restless teen in the film
Disturbia, the exciting beatnik era was the latest buzz—much like coffee plants in places like Brazil and Colombia. It was cool to hang out at
coffeehouses, places to talk, read poetry—and savor coffee, the beverage that stimulates the mind. Men and women sipped coffee, espresso,
and cappuccino and they wore black turtlenecks, sunglasses, and
skinny black pants. I was too young to be a big part of the Beat era but
old enough to know it existed.

One Friday after school when walking home from school, I passed
the house rented by a group of beatniks. I walked up to the front door.
It was quiet. My eyes feasted through the windows to see a kitchen
and living room chock-full of books, pillows, low tables, and mis-
matched empty coffee cups on top. I opened the door and a wicker
chest was in the hallway, sitting there like Pandora's Box. I opened it,
inch by inch. I was greeted by wine bottles. It made sense that countless coffee cups were a household tool to sober up. While I learned
during my wonder years that coffee played a role in my life as I knew it,

it wasn't until later that I discovered how important the coffee bean was around the globe.

In the 21st century, I believe it's a diet of Mother Nature's finest superfoods that is key to keeping healthy and staving off heart disease, high blood pressure, type 2 diabetes—and obesity. And yes! Yes, coffee can and does help fight and even prevent health problems. Here's the ongoing health buzz about healing coffee.

SO, HOW DOES COFFEE HEAL, ANYHOW?

While coffee types have different healing properties, coffee itself has many healing powers. It's the antioxidants: These enzymes work both inside the body and outside the body to help stave off disease. And there is so much more. . . .

Since the beginning of a goatherd and his dancing goats that enjoyed the perks of coffee berries, coffee has proved its worth in stimulating both body and mind for centuries. However, in the 20th century, coffee got a bad reputation and the idea of this popular "drug" as a health food was unbelievable.

Then, much like dark chocolate, a wave of studies around the world changed the mindset of doctors and scientists. Coffee, the beverage that folks still love, good or bad, has shown in stacks of studies that it may do more than get you up when the alarm goes off.

Thanks to the researchers who think outside of the box and inside the bag or can of coffee, we now know America's favorite beverage can lower rates of life-threatening diseases. That cup of coffee may stave off cancer, heart disease, type 2 diabetes, and more. The consensus is coffee—yes, coffee—can be good for your health.

In the 21st century, the buzz is—coffee heals. Past and present-day studies (not just "rat approved") in the United States and other countries, too, point to the healing powers of coffee. Here, take a sobering peek at what's going on in the world of coffee and health.

COFFEE AND THE BIG C

Cancer is a frightening disease. Nobody is immune. The upside is, many types of cancers if caught in time can be treated and life goes on. For decades I've been writing about anticancer foods and lifestyle changes that may help keep cancers at bay. And now, amazingly, coffee, which has gotten a bad rap in the past, is getting kudos for its role in beating the battle of the Big C.

How Coffee Works: Researchers are quick to point out cancer-fighting antioxidants (in both caffeinated and decaf), which may help lower the risk of developing some cancers, including breast, prostate, and liver.

Breast Cancer. Can coffee lower the risk of developing breast cancer? The answer may be "yes," and postmenopausal women, like me, are welcoming the exciting news. A study published online in the journal *Breast Cancer Research* analyzed findings of almost 6,000 postmenopausal Swedish women aged 50 to 74 and discovered heavy coffee drinkers had a lower risk of developing estrogen receptor-negative breast cancer. Credit may be due to the fact that coffee raises blood levels of a phytochemical that has been linked with a lower risk of this estrogen-related breast cancer.[2]

Cheryl Norman, 62, never drank coffee in her life until she finished her breast cancer treatment. "Diet Coke was my beverage of choice," she recalls. "Thanks to chemo, I now can't stand the taste of colas." So, she turned to gourmet flavored coffees as a treat. "When I read coffee contains an ingredient that helps suppress estrogen (and since I take meds for that), I figured why not."

Liver Cancer. More good news about coffee and cancer shows that daily coffee drinkers may also be protecting themselves from liver cancer. It may be the antioxidants in coffee that shield the liver from the bad effects of carcinogens (cancer-causing compounds). And caffeine is not to be left out, either, since it may be another piece of the anti-cancer puzzle. "In August 2007, the journal *Hepatology*, reported that 10 different studies, conducted in Europe and Japan, showed that people who drink coffee have a significantly reduced chance of developing liver cancer. The studies included about 240,000 people, including 2,260 suffering from liver cancer, and showed that people who drank at least several cups of coffee every day had less than half the chance of being diagnosed with liver cancer than study participants who drank no coffee—the odds dropped by 23 percent with each daily cup. . . . There is some speculation that coffee causes liver enzymes to become stronger," explains the *Dr. Chopra Says* authors in their book, which may prevent liver scarring, reducing the risk of developing liver cancer. And that's not all.[3]

Oral Cancer. Liver cancer is deadly, as is oral cancer, especially when it's not detected in early stages. University of Milan researchers discovered that more than 14,000 people who drank more than four cups of coffee each day have 39 percent lower odds of getting mouth or throat cancer than people who did not drink java. And there's more. It's not the caffeine, say the Italian scientists, pointing out that coffee contains more than 1,000 chemicals, including the anticancer compounds cafestol and kahweol.[4]

Prostate Cancer. I've never met a man who doesn't like coffee. Sadly, I have known men who have fallen victim to prostate cancer and didn't survive. The upside: Researchers from the Harvard School of Public Health discovered men who drank the most coffee—regular or decaf—have the least risk for prostate cancer, noted in a study for more than a decade. Approximately 50,000 U.S. men reported their coffee intake every four years from 1986 to 2008. The evidence revealed that coffee was linked with lower risk of prostate cancer, liver cancer, and other diseases, too.

Men who drank six cups or more per day had a whopping 60 percent lower risk of developing deadly prostate cancer, and 20 percent lower risk of developing any form of the disease, outlined the study published in the online edition of the *Journal of the National Cancer Institute.* But even drinking a more normal amount, such as up to three cups, was linked with a 30 percent lower risk of lethal prostate cancer.

It didn't matter if the guys sipped regular or decaf—the caffeine jolt wasn't key. Instead, the protection may be connected to the other compounds in coffee, such as antioxidants, reducing inflammation and regulating insulin.[5]

Skin Cancer. Recent research, published in *Proceedings of the National Academy of Sciences,* shows that caffeine may guard against skin cancer, the most common cancer in the United States, according to the American Cancer Society. Rutgers and University of Washington researchers found caffeine changes the activity of a gene involved in the destruction of cells with DNA damage. The findings: Rodents given caffeinated water had 70 percent fewer tumors—perhaps because caffeine acts as a sunscreen.[6]

What You Can Do: No man or woman can live on coffee alone, but research is piling up showing that it's good for you, and countless people cannot see living life without it. Also, eating fruits and vegetables, staying lean, exercising, and having preventive cancer screenings can help keep cancer out of your life. And superfood coffee—the organic, medium-roast-antioxidant-rich types—paired with anticancer superfoods can be the beginning of an arsenal for you to keep the Big C out of your life.

HEART LIFESAVER

Once again, I sit here noting the American Heart Association's observation that heart disease is still America's number one killer for both men and women. These days, however, coffee consumption is not to be excluded in heart health—and there are many reasons why this fact will win the hearts of devout coffee lovers, like me—and perhaps you, too. Here is the buzz on coffee and your heart.

High Blood Pressure

First of all, the old school says that drinking coffee, especially because of its caffeine content, can create a quick spike in your blood pressure numbers—both systolic and diastolic. However, there is controversy about caffeine's effect on blood pressure.

As a Type A individual who is constantly at work to keep her BP numbers low, I wanted to see if drinking a cup of java would instantly cause my blood pressure to rise. To my surprise, time after time, it lowered the numbers. It actually calms me. It's believed by nutritionists that for people who do not normally consume caffeinated coffee often they may see a spike in their BP numbers versus people who drink a cup of java on a regular basis—like I do.

The 150 Healthiest Foods on Earth author Jonny Bowden, Ph.D., writes about a 12-year study by Harvard researchers of 155,000 women (published in the November 9, 2005, issue of the *Journal of the American Medical Association*). The findings were that drinking caffeinated cola may be associated with an increased risk of high blood pressure, but the same problem was *not* found with caffeinated coffee. Actually, the study suggested that women who drink caffeinated coffee may actually have a *reduced risk* of high blood pressure. That said, Bowden claims "there's no good reason to forego reasonable amounts of coffee unless, of course, you have a medical condition like hypertension, in which case coffee is probably *not* a good idea."[7]

I sip and savor no more than 12 ounces of coffee daily, and when I do milk is definitely part of the beverage. Plus, the java jolt provides me with energy to walk the dogs, swim, and stay physical throughout the day.

How Coffee Works: It's believed by some doctors that some people, perhaps like me, who drink caffeinated beverages, including coffee, build up a tolerance to it. This, in turn, means caffeine doesn't have a long-term effect on my blood pressure. Also, after I exercise, I notice my BP reading is low—just like after drinking coffee. Could it be the endorphin feel-good natural high that provides a sense of well-being and normal blood pressure?

What You Can Do: Try drinking less rather than more coffee, but enjoy a quality brew. Limit your caffeine intake to approximately 200 to 300 milligrams per day. Pairing coffee beverages with milk and/or honey will increase the odds of you getting your antioxidants, minerals, and other good-for-you compounds—and if you don't overindulge but keep physical and lean (refer to chapter 10, "The Skinny Beverage")—those BP numbers at 120/80 (or less) and your heart rate at 60 should be a goal you can reach and maintain.

And chances are, if coffee in moderation is working for your BP levels, it may help keep your cholesterol in check, too.

Cholesterol Ups and Downs

In adults, total cholesterol levels of 240 milligrams or higher are in the high risk territory and levels from 200 to 239 are considered borderline high risk. Triglycerides should not be more than 150. Research proves that antioxidants—like the kind found in that mug of morning coffee or java during a coffee break—can help you stay heart healthy.

How Coffee Works: Because coffee (hold the sugar and cream) may help you to lose unwanted extra weight and motivate you to exercise it could help to boost cholesterol numbers and lower bad cholesterol. Caveat: If you have high cholesterol, it may be due to your mom or dad and coffee won't be the quick fix for you.

What You Can Do: Also, it is filtered coffee that is cholesterol friendly—not the unfiltered coffee brew method, which may up cholesterol numbers. Some scientists are pinpointing unfiltered coffee that you should be concerned about, especially if high cholesterol is a genetic factor for you or you're fighting to keep the numbers in check.

It's boiled coffee—grounds combined with boiling water and steeped—like espresso, plunger pot coffee, and Turkish coffee, that presents the biggest risks. It's not the caffeine, either. Blame the two cholesterol-causing compounds called cafestol and kahweol (but ironically they help fight cancer).[8]

Keep coffee in perspective, though. If you're sedentary, smoke, and eat a high-cholesterol diet—these factors probably wreak more havoc on your blood cholesterol than a cup or two of unfiltered java. While filtered coffee in moderation may lower your risk of developing heart disease, it is the wholesome diet and lifestyle habits (including regular exercise) that can also help you regulate cholesterol levels and blood pressure and keep heart problems at bay—and don't forget the scourge of diabetes.

COFFEE AND DIABETES

Medical doctors know and you, like me, may know through friends or family that type 2 diabetes continues to rise in the United States. Researchers at the Harvard School of Public Health and Brigham and Women's Hospital studied 125,000 people from 1980 to 1998—and discovered a shocking benefit of coffee: People who drink coffee on a regular basis can significantly lower their risk of type 2 diabetes. The findings were promising: "Men who drank six or more cups of caffeinated coffee daily reduced their risk for this terrible disease by 50 percent; women who drank the same amount reduced their risk by 30 percent," write the authors of *Doctor Chopra Says*.[9]

How Coffee Works: Researchers will tell you that coffee's power as a diabetes remedy may not be due to only caffeine but also to its other components, including chlorogenic acids, lignans, and magnesium, which also may be part of the package that can help keep type 2 diabetes at bay.

Adds antioxidant guru Dr. Joe Vinson, coffee is good to prevent diabetes "but not good if you have prediabetes or diabetes, because the caffeine overcomes the antioxidants' effect on glucose and insulin. Decaf coffee is preferred for those people, as they will still get some antioxidants."

What You Can Do: Try to limit coffee intake to two to three cups per day. Also, eating more fiber-rich foods, lowering dietary fat, and exercising regularly helps aid in sugar blood control. People who have type 2 diabetes can usually control the disease by diet and lifestyle changes. To be safe, always check with your health-care provider before making any sweet changes to your daily regime.

This recipe is chock-full of superfoods, including garlic, onions, vinegar, lemon juice, and coffee. It's foods like these, as well as fish, chicken, and chops, that are part of the Mediterranean heart-healthy diet.

BBQ Sauce
❖ ❖ ❖

2–3 pounds of raw chicken for barbecuing
2 cloves crushed garlic
½ cup molasses
¼ cup lemon juice
1½ tablespoons dry mustard
½ cup brown sugar
¼ cup Worcestershire sauce
Salt and pepper to taste

1 cup finely chopped onions
1 cup chopped bell pepper
1 cup catsup
1 tablespoon or taste Tabasco sauce
¼ cup white vinegar
½ cup your favorite blend brewed Chock full o'Nuts coffee

Combine all ingredients in a large saucepan. Bring to a boil. Stirring constantly, reduce heat and simmer until onions and bell pepper are very tender, about 1 hour. Let cool. Marinate chicken pieces in sauce for at least 4 hours, ideally overnight. Also great on shrimp and chops.

(*Courtesy:* Chock full o'Nuts.)

In the next chapter, your eyebrows will rise, like mine did, when you find out that coffee is left out (sort of) of the Mediterranean Diet. That being said, I discovered that Oldways Preservation & Exchange Trust does give the drink enjoyed in Mediterranean countries credit. After all, it's the antideprivation eating and lifestyle habits in European countries—regular exercise teamed with enjoying a coffee break on a daily basis—that have been part of the past and present and most likely will be part of the future. Not to forget many coffee beverages were derived and are still appreciated in Italy, France, and many other Mediterranean countries.

A CUP FULL OF PERKS

✓ Coffee may help boost your quality of life and stave off life-threatening diseases.

✓ Healing coffee and its powers are acknowledged around the world in studies as a healing medicine.

✓ Stacks of studies, past and present, show that regular coffee drinkers may help lower their risk of developing diseases, including cancers, heart disease, and diabetes, and other ailments that can up the odds of being one more statistic.

✓ Coffee is healthful in a variety of ways—and credit is due to the variety of disease-fighting antioxidants, caffeine, and other compounds.

COFFEE KEEPS THE DOCTOR AWAY

Disease	How Coffee Works
Heart Disease	Antioxidants in coffee help to lower the risk of high blood pressure, high cholesterol.
Diabetes	Coffee may lower the insulin and the risk of developing type 2 diabetes.
Cancer	Antioxidants in coffee act as disease-fighting antioxidants to hinder the cancer process and may reduce certain cancers, including breast, prostate, and liver.

The Mediterranean Cuppa Comfort

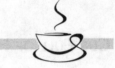

Strong coffee, much strong coffee, is what awakens me. Coffee gives me warmth, waking, an unusual force and a pain that is not without very great pleasure.

—Napoleon Bonaparte[1]

When I was 16, my family uprooted me to a city-type home without an outdoorsy environment. Like a desperate coffee tree amid pests and a drought, I didn't adapt. I rebelled and reunited with trees. My first hitchhiking trip was on a cloudy fall Sunday afternoon. I departed from San Jose to Los Gatos, a town with coffee shops. I ordered a to-go coffee with equal portions of hot chocolate (like the Swiss do)—and stood on the roadside waiting for a ride. Before I finished my warm, chocolaty drink, I was on my way on Highway 9, a mountain paradise, to Santa Cruz, a beach town. And the caffeine jolt made the waiting for rides and conversation with strangers more stimulating.

I ended up at the Catalysts, a happening coffee shop, filled with down-to-earth locals. The shop's blackboard offered a wide world of types of coffee. It was the dark roasts—Italian and French—that had me at first sight. But I ended up ordering a safe cinnamon light roast.

It was the start of a journey of soul-searching and the coffee buzz titillated my thoughts, dreams, and uplifted my spirit. And while sipping a cup of java I ordered a pastry. I spoke to strangers and the dangling conversations made me feel alive like bright red coffee berries on a tree.

And while I didn't know it then, later on as a health author I learned I was enjoying both forbidden coffee and decadent chocolate—foods of the Mediterranean diet for the comfort of it all.

COFFEE MANIA IN THE MEDITERRANEAN

In the *Healing Powers* book series, I tout the Mediterranean diet, time after time. The diet and lifestyle go back in time to the traditional diet eaten by people in Crete. Back in the day when I was born, and throughout the sixties, the Mediterranean diet was believed to be connected to healthy life—and this has not changed in the 21st century. A plant-based-foods diet—full of fruits and vegetables but also consisting of whole grains, beans, legumes, nuts and seeds, and olive oil—has been proven to lower the risk of heart disease, diabetes, and obesity.

But surprisingly, you won't see coffee included in the Oldways traditional Mediterranean diet pyramid. It is not part of Mediterranean diet. (But you will see drinking water—which a cup of coffee does give you—is included.)

So I asked the good people at Oldways, "Why isn't coffee included in the Mediterranean Diet Pyramid?" The answer was interesting, confirming that they do not say the word "coffee" in any of the literature about the Mediterranean diet. I was told by the staff point-blank that although there is a lot in the literature about the healthful nature of coffee, it is more disease specific: "K. Dun Gifford, president of Oldways, tried to get the scientists to include coffee with the pyramid (because everyone in the Mediterranean really does drink coffee—11:00 A.M. in Italy means it's time to nudge up to the coffee bar for an espresso), but Dun could never get total agreement from the scientists, so we cannot use it on the pyramid."

But Oldways did go the extra mile for giving coffee due credit. In 2006 Oldways compiled an impressive booklet, *Coffee and Health: An Educational Program "Refreshingly Good News for Coffee Lovers"* (subsidized by Dunkin' Donuts), and held a seminar to discuss the benefits of coffee.

Gifford wrote: "We drink coffee to wake up, to stay up, and to sober up. We drink it steaming hot and iced cold; black and blonde; bitter and sweet. We stir it with cinnamon sticks and add brandy to it. We sweeten and enrich it with sugar, cream, ice cream, chocolate and no-cal sweeteners. We flavor it with vanilla, raspberries, and dozens more flavorings. We steam it to make cappuccino and concoct dozens of variants. We cook and bake with it, too."[2]

Added the coffee-savvy Oldways president: "Finns, Swedes, Danes drink nearly three times as much coffee as we Americans do; Germans and Austrians drink about twice as much; French and Swiss a bit more; and Italians and Colombians about the same as we Americans."[3]

So, while coffee isn't technically an image on the Oldways traditional Mediterranean diet pyramid, people who live in Mediterranean countries—as well as people behind Oldways—know all too well that coffee has a place in the hearts of Mediterranean people and the lifestyle, past and present.

CAFÉ ROOTS ARE MEDITERRANEAN

If you go to Europe, you won't have to go far to see coffee everywhere you go. The popular beverage is available in coffee bars, bistros, coffeehouses—both in Western and Eastern Europe. Here, take a peek at the roots of coffee from yesteryear.

1. The first Parisian café opened in 1689.
2. In the year 1763, there were over 200 coffee shops in Venice.
3. The prototype of the first espresso machine was created in France in 1822.
4. The average age of an Italian barista is 48. "Barista" is a respected job title in Italy.
5. Italians do not drink espresso during meals. It is considered to be a separate event and given its own time.
6. In Italy, espresso is considered so essential to daily life that the price is regulated by the government.
7. Italy now has over 200,000 coffee bars, and the number is still growing.

8. "Latte" is the Italian word for milk. So if you request a latte in Italy, you'll be served a glass of milk.
9. The year was 1716 when Venetian coffee shop merchants began distributing leaflets exalting their new product: coffee. This may be the first example of advertising for coffee shops.
10. In the later part of the 1600s, a café in Venice began serving beverages made from water and ice. It also served roasted coffee.[4]

PAIRING COFFEE AND MEDITERRANEAN DIET SUPERFOODS

In my *Healing Powers* book series I push the philosophy that there is no one quick fix for good health by eating one superfood—including vinegar, olive oil, or chocolate. Not only would it be a boring way to eat, but it's the total package of the versatile traditional Mediterranean diet and lifestyle that is a path to good health. Welcome to my world, where I abide by the New Coffee Rules I incorporated into my Mediterranean diet regime.

COFFEE RULE #1: Going vegan: I eat a plant-based diet, including fruits and vegetables, wholes grains, nuts, and seeds. **A Spoonful of Espresso:** Try savoring a cup of espresso or a chocolate- or nut-flavored coffee before or after eating a meal including these vegan foods.

COFFEE RULE #2: Eating fresh foods: If it's fresh I'm there with open hands, and this rule includes finding a coffee roaster. **A Spoonful of Espresso:** I include exotic coffees in my diet and lifestyle.

COFFEE RULE #3: Using coffee like an Italian: I use coffee in many forms in cooking and baking. **A Spoonful of Joe:** I sometimes use espresso powder in smoothies and shakes to give them a java kick.

COFFEE RULE #4: Kissing off saturated fat: I aim for a daily total fat amount ranging from about 25 to 35 percent of energy, with saturated fat composing no more than 7 to 8 percent of calories. It's easier to do when you stay clear of coffee flavorings, including whole milk

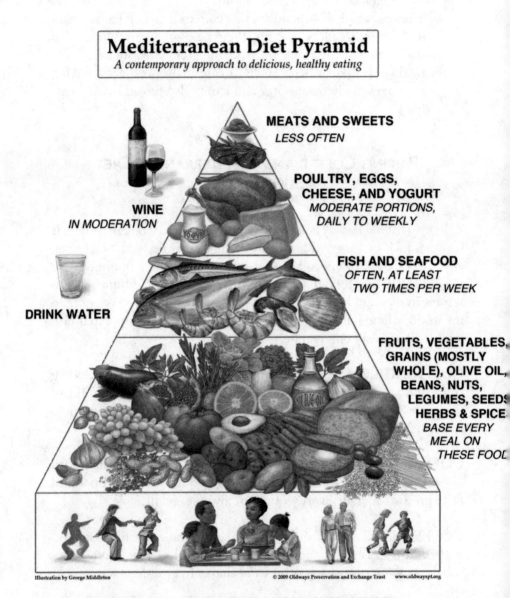

Mediterranean Diet Pyramid
A contemporary approach to delicious, healthy eating

MEATS AND SWEETS
LESS OFTEN

POULTRY, EGGS, CHEESE, AND YOGURT
MODERATE PORTIONS, DAILY TO WEEKLY

WINE
IN MODERATION

FISH AND SEAFOOD
OFTEN, AT LEAST TWO TIMES PER WEEK

DRINK WATER

FRUITS, VEGETABLES, GRAINS (MOSTLY WHOLE), OLIVE OIL, BEANS, NUTS, LEGUMES, SEEDS HERBS & SPICE
BASE EVERY MEAL ON THESE FOOD

Illustration by George Middleton

© 2009 Oldways Preservation and Exchange Trust   www.oldwayspt.org

BE PHYSICALLY ACTIVE; ENJOY MEALS WITH OTHERS

and creamers. **A Spoonful of Joe:** Adding natural flavor such as cinnamon or cocoa powder can enhance a cup of coffee without the fat.

COFFEE RULE #5: Including cheese and yogurt: No need to stay clear of goat cheese, Greek yogurt, and coffee can be part of it. **A Spoonful of Joe:** Instead of eating fruit yogurt infused with artificial fruits and sweeteners, I've grown to love all-natural Greek yogurt with a sprinkle of espresso powder.

COFFEE RULE #6: Eating lean protein: I include fish (such as wild salmon and water-packed tuna) and poultry (chicken and turkey), with an iced or hot coffee beverage after. **A Spoonful of Joe:** I have also tried adding espresso powder to sauces (low fat like marinara) and basting them on fish and poultry.

COFFEE RULE #7: Savoring natural desserts: I lean toward fresh fruit as my daily dessert and limit sweets (except for flavored coffees). **A Spoonful of Joe:** Two cups of coffee per day is my limit. Savoring espresso drinks, including a cappuccino and café au lait, helps to keep my calories in check because these are special treats teamed with calcium-rich milk. I rarely add syrups and sugar. Once you learn to enjoy an excellent cup of java, a splash of organic milk is all you'll need. Cravings for high-fat, sugary decadent desserts subside, and when you do give in it will be guilt free. You'll be feeding your sweet tooth in moderation.

COFFEE RULE #8: Avoiding red meat: The truth is, I haven't touched meat for more than 30 years. The Mediterranean diet allows lean meat a few times per month—but I avoid it to keep lean like a carnivorous cat. **A Spoonful of Joe:** Refer to rule #6 and try espresso in sauces on lean meat dishes with plenty of fresh, seasonal vegetables.

COFFEE RULE #9: Enjoying regular exercise: I swim and walk my dogs to keep my weight and blood pressure in check, stay fit, and feel energized. **A Spoonful of Joe:** Drinking a cup of coffee, whether it is an espresso-spiked Americano or frappe (also known as a latte granita), before walking the dogs or going swimming gives me an extra oomph and intensifies my concentration on walking farther or swimming better and more laps. It's a feel-good physical trainer.

COFFEE RULE #10: Drinking wine: Red wine is heart healthy, but coffee before or after can give you antioxidants, too. A Spoonful of Joe: There are scrumptious coffee drinks that do include alcohol. Flavored Colombian coffees with yummy artificial liquors are enough for me to get a buzz and stay sober and happy.

Using the Coffee Rules, teaming foods and flavors of the Mediterranean diet (as shown in the chart) with coffee is a good way to eat and a good path to good health.

ETHNIC CUISINE, COFFEE CHOICES

Like Europeans, I enjoy eating a variety of common Mediterranean foods and getting daily physical activity. It's this diet and lifestyle that works to lower your risk of developing diseases and ups your odds of living a longer, quality life whether you reside in Europe or America. If you can't whisk away to another country and enjoy exotic foods, you certainly can bring a taste of another place to you. Pairing ethnic cuisines and coffees from different regions is an excellent way to experience a great escape in the comfort of your home. Here, take a look.

Chinese Cuisine: Traditional Chinese food can be healthful—low-fat and low-cal. Translation: Opt for rice, veggies, and seafood. Best Picks: chop suey, moo goo gai pan, steamed dumplings, steamed white rice, stir-fried seafood and vegetables, and steamed vegetables. *Coffee Choice:* Kona, flavored with spices.

French Cuisine: This cuisine can be fattening, but it doesn't have to be. Instead of diving into sauces made with cream and butter, you can go the leaner route. Best Picks: endive and watercress greens (use olive oil and red wine vinegar dressing), sautéed vegetables, chicken in wine sauce, French bread drizzled with olive oil, and fresh fruit. *Coffee Choice:* French Roast, espresso.

Italian Cuisine: Pasta and pizza—these foods can be oh so fattening, but they don't have to be. Think whole-grain pasta with marinara sauce and thin-crust vegetarian pizza and you'll do fine with taste and not fat overload. Best Picks: tomato-based soups, chicken cacciatore, fresh fruit. *Coffee Choice:* cappuccino with skim milk, Italian Roast.

Common Foods and Flavors of the Mediterranean Diet Pyramid

Vegetables & Tubers	Artichokes, Arugula, Beets, Broccoli, Brussels Sprouts, Cabbage, Carrots, Celery, Celeriac, Chicory, Collard Cucumber, Dandelion Greens, Eggplant, Fennel, Kale, Leeks, Lettuce, Mache, Mushrooms, Mustard Greens, Nettles, Okra, Onions (red, sweet, white), Peas, Peppers, Potatoes, Pumpkin, Purslane, Radishes, Rutabega, Scallions, Shallots, Spinach, Sweet Potatoes, Turnips, Zucchini
Fruits	Avocados, Apples, Apricots, Cherries, Clementines, Dates, Figs, Grapefruit, Grapes, Lemons, Oranges, Melons, Nectarines, Olives, Peaches, Pears, Pomegranates, Strawberries, Tangerines, Tomatoes
Grains	Breads, Barley, Buckwheat, Bulgur, Couscous, Durum, Farro, Millet, Oats, Polenta, Rice, Wheatberries
Fish & Seafood	Abalone, Cockles, Clams, Crab, Eel, Flounder, Lobster, Mackerel, Mussels, Octopus, Oysters, Salmon, Sardines, Sea Bass, Shrimp, Squid, Tilapia, Tuna, Whelk, Yellowtail
Poultry, Eggs, Cheese, & Yogurt	Chicken, Duck, Guinea Fowl Eggs (Chicken, Quail, and Duck) Cheeses (Examples Include: Brie, Chevre, Corvo, Feta, Haloumi, Manchego, Parmigiano-Reggiano, Pecorino, Ricotta) Yogurt, Greek Yogurt
Nuts, Seeds, & Legumes	Almonds, Beans (Cannellini, Chickpeas, Fava, Kidney, Green), Cashews, Hazelnuts, Lentils, Pine Nuts, Pistachios, Sesame Seeds (Tahini), Split Peas, Walnuts
Herbs & Spices	Anise, Basil, Bay Leaf, Chiles, Clove, Cumin, Fennel, Garlic, Lavender, Marjoram, Mint, Oregano, Parsley, Pepper, Pul Biber, Rosemary, Sage, Savory, Sumac, Tarragon, Thyme, Za'atar
Meats & Sweets	Pork, Beef, Lamb, Mutton, Goat Sweets (Examples include: Baklava, Biscotti, Crème Caramel, Chocolate, Gelato, Fruit Tarts, Kunefe, Lokum, Mousse Au Chocolat, Sorbet, Tiramisu)
Water & Wine	Drink Plenty of Water Wine in Moderation

www.oldwayspt.org

Indian Cuisine: This type of food can be healthy and lean with its poultry, rice, and vegetables—and stay away from dishes served with peanut sauce, fried turnovers and fritters, and cream soups. Best Picks: bean dishes, tandoori chicken and fish, pita-type bread, chicken kabobs, and yogurt cucumber salad can make you feel like you're in India without racking up unwanted calories or fat. *Coffee Choice:* Java, Mocha Java.

Mexican Cuisine: Traditional Mexican fare can be fattening, but it doesn't have to be. If you stick with fajitas, soft tacos, burritos and salads, chicken and salsa, and less rather than more cheese you'll do fine. Best Picks: chicken soft tacos, chicken and vegetable fajitas, corn tortillas with salsa, a taco salad with vegetables and salsa. *Coffee Choice:* Guatemalan, Colombian.

Okay, so coffee is savored and paired with many cuisines in the Mediterranean countries—and other regions, too. It's not just me and the people behind Oldways who know coffee is prized in Europe and around the world. Actually, many of the foods in the Mediterranean diet go with coffee like honey goes with tea. This biscotti recipe is for an Italian cookie that is perfect dipped in your favorite cup of coffee, wherever you are or wherever you want to feel like you should be.

Barista Biscotti Bites

❖ ❖ ❖

BISCOTTI

6 tablespoons (3 ounces) butter

⅔ cup (5 ounces) brown sugar, packed

¼ teaspoon salt

¼ teaspoon hazelnut flavor or 1 teaspoon vanilla extract

1 teaspoon espresso powder

1½ teaspoons baking powder

2 large eggs

2 cups (8½ ounces) King Arthur Unbleached All-Purpose Flour

1 cup (7 ounces) cappuccino chips*

CHOCOLATE GANACHE

1 cup (6 ounces) chopped
  semi-sweet chocolate
  or chocolate chips
1/3 cup (2⅝ ounces) half-
  and-half

¼ teaspoon espresso
  powder
⅛ teaspoon hazelnut flavor

Preheat the oven to 350°F. Lightly grease (or line with parchment) one large (about 18-by-13-inch) baking sheet.

In a medium-sized bowl, beat the butter, sugar, salt, flavor or extract, espresso powder, and baking powder until the mixture is smooth and creamy. Beat in the eggs; the batter may look slightly curdled. At the low speed of your mixer, add the flour and chips, stirring until smooth; the dough will be sticky.

Divide the dough in half, plopping each half onto the prepared baking sheet. Using your wet fingers, shape each piece into a rough log about 12 inches long, 2 inches wide, and about ¾ inch thick. Straighten the log, and smooth its top and sides.

Bake the dough for 25 minutes. Remove it from the oven, and allow it to cool in the pan anywhere from 10 to 25 minutes; just work it into the schedule of whatever else you're doing in the kitchen. Using a spray bottle filled with room-temperature water, lightly but thoroughly spritz the logs, making sure to cover the sides as well as the top. Softening the crust just this little bit will make slicing the biscotti much easier.

Reduce the oven temperature to 325°F. Wait another 5 minutes, then use a serrated knife to cut the log crosswise into ½" to ¾" slices. As you're slicing, be sure to cut straight up and down, perpendicular to the pan; if you cut unevenly, biscotti may be thicker at the top than the bottom and they'll topple over during their second bake.

Set the biscotti on the edge of the prepared baking sheet. Return the biscotti to the oven and bake them for 25 to 30 minutes, till they feel very dry. They'll still feel a

*Hazelnut flavor and creamy, coffee-flavored cappuccino chips are key elements in the flavor of these biscotti. However, substitute vanilla extract and white chocolate or semi-sweet chips if you like.

tiny bit moist in the very center, if you break off a piece; but they'll continue to dry out as they cool. Remove the biscotti from the oven, and transfer them to a rack to cool.

To Make the Ganache

Combine the chocolate and half-and-half in a microwave-safe bowl, and heat for about 45 seconds, or until the cream is very hot. Stir until the chocolate melts and the mixture is smooth and creamy, reheating briefly if necessary. Stir in the espresso powder and hazelnut flavor.

Dip about ½ of each biscotti in the ganache. Lay dipped biscotti on a piece of parchment that you've sprayed with non-stick spray; a piece of waxed paper; or a cooling rack. Allow biscotti to harden for several hours or overnight before wrapping for storage. Yield: 3 dozen 3½-inch biscotti.

(*Courtesy:* King Arthur Flour.)

While biscotti pairs well with coffee, different types of roasts teamed with other ingredients have medicinal properties. Take a look at part 3, "Healing Coffees," to see the wide, wide world of coffees and you, like me, can enjoy coffee with amazing flavor around the globe without taking a vacation.

A Cup Full of Perks

✓ Coffee has made its mark in the past in the Mediterranean countries, in the cities of Paris and Venice, and the nation of Italy and has held its place in the present day.

✓ The Oldways traditional Mediterranean diet pyramid doesn't include coffee, but the organization praises coffee's versatile virtues.

✓ Teaming European-based espresso with Mediterranean foods is a wonderful way to get a taste of the Old World ...

✓ ... And by pairing coffee with other ethnic cuisines, whether it is Mexican fare or eats from India, you'll get health benefits of a variety of foods and treat your palate.

PART 3

HEALING COFFEES

Types of Blends and Roasts

*Coffee: Induces wit. Good only if it comes through
Havre. After a big dinner party it is taken standing
up. Take it without sugar—very swank: gives the
impression you have lived in the East.*
—Gustave Flaubert (1821–1880)[1]

After my short trips enhanced with coffee breaks, bicycling trips
teamed with coffee followed. At 18, I enrolled in junior college. I met
a fellow student who taught me how to eat right and be more physically active—like traditional Europeans. We were both physical education majors. Riding ten speeds to and from campus—with the help of
coffee and other exercise, it changed my life as I once knew it. I ate
only nutrient-dense foods and sipped black coffee in between our
never-ending on-the-road adventures, which were a great escape from
school and home.

One night, buzzed on coffee, we rode for miles, to parks and parties.
We ended up at an apartment complex and met two male fellow students. We ended up swimming in the pool with them under the
moonlight, complete with chicken fights. And after our child-like play,
my friend and I got warm and cozy inside our male friends' apartment.
Instead of plain fresh-brewed coffee, we were served a flavored espresso
drink with steamed milk and chocolate syrup. It was my first taste of a
mocha cappuccino. (I discovered later that the word "cappuccino" is

linked to the brown and white cowl worn by monks in Italy.) The flavor of the caffeinated beverage enhanced the night of enjoying lingering conversation until dawn.

Coffee lovers of all ages around the nation have discovered, like I did, the physical and mental stimulation enhanced by coffee. Different types of coffees from different locations around the globe can make a difference, too. Besides location, other factors come into play of the quality and flavor of coffee.

HOT COFFEES FROM COOL COUNTRIES

While there are dozens of varietals of coffee in the United States, as I noted earlier, it's believed by coffee proponents that there may be hundreds more around the globe. If you're craving a trip or foods from a faraway foreign country, you can get a taste of exciting tastes and textures without getting on an airplane. Just turn to a coffee of the region and pair it with cuisine.

At least once a month during my trip to Coffee World, I would find a box of coffee bags—from Colombia, Guatemala, Brazil, and Hawaii—on my doorstep. Many of these coffees come from giant coffee companies and smaller coffee roasters, too. And it was a dream come true to be able to taste these delights.

LET'S GO CUPPIN'

Cupping is a way to judge coffee quality. So industry professionals taste wine, olive oil, chocolate, and honey. And yes, coffee is judged for its flavor, too. The technical term is "cupping," and it lets the coffee be tasted. The cupper—a pro or you—"slurps" a spoonful with a sniff. Coffee is judged for its characteristics and imperfections but also for its blending, beans, and roast. There are so many coffee types to taste, where do you begin?

There are so many types of coffee in the Coffee World, I'm feeling like Tom Hanks's character's statement in the film *You've Got Mail:* "The whole purpose of places like Starbucks is for people with no decision-making ability whatsoever to make six decisions just to buy one cup of coffee. Short, tall, light, dark, caf, decaf, lowfat, non-fat, etcetera. So people who don't know what the hell they're doing or who on earth they are can, for only $2.95, get not just a cup of coffee but an absolutely defining sense of self: Tall. Decaf. Cappuccino." And while these are some choices to make, there are so many more to make when it comes to types of coffees. Here, take a look at several that will take your breath away.

POPULAR TASTING TERMS: THE BREW

The Bad	The Good
Acidity: Bright, tangy, fruity or wine-like flavor characteristics found in many high-grown arabica coffees; acidity is reduced as coffee is roasted darker	**Body:** Full-bodied coffees have a strong, creamy, and pleasant mouthful
Astringent: A dry, sour, salty taste	**Bright:** Pleasant, almost tangy flavor
Bitter: Harsh, unpleasant taste; bitterness of overextracted, defective, dark-roasted coffees	**Clean:** Flavorful, but without any pungent flavors
Briny: A salty taste caused by continuously heating coffee after brewing is complete	**Mellow:** Balanced and mild, without strong tastes or aftertastes; medium roasted
Ferment: A sour and oniony taste over fermented coffee	**Neutral:** Doesn't have a a predominant taste; used in blending
Flat: Lacking flavor or aroma	**Smooth:** A taste of balance without aftertastes
Harsh: Pungent, such as low-quality, bitter robusta	

(*Courtesy:* Zecuppa Coffee, LLC.)

COFFEES FROM AROUND THE WORLD

Here are just a few coffee types that you'll find noteworthy, from country to country, in the bean belt around the globe. I'm adding a sweet treat (either fruit or chocolate) that pairs well with each coffee from each region.

The Americas: North America and the Caribbean

Hawaii: Though coffee farms are found throughout the Hawaiian Islands, it is Kona coffee from the large island of Hawaii that is best known and always in demand. Hawaiian coffee is carefully processed and produces a deliciously rich, aromatic cup of medium body. The first time I traveled to the Big Island, I was greeted with a decadent breakfast to love. The cheese omelet, toast, and fresh orange juice in the outdoor café environment were memorable, but the coffee was smooth and rich while I sipped it in the company of wild birds and fragrant flowers. Sweet Treat: Angel cake.

Hawaiian Coffees

At first glance, the Hawaiian Islands with their fertile valleys and lush forests seem a virtual paradise. They have long been thought of as a haven for creatures of all kinds. But Hawaii is also known as coffee paradise.

More than 25 years ago, I was introduced to my first bag of genuine Kona coffee. It was a Christmas gift from my sister who lives on the Big Island. Inside the brown box were a sealed bag of coffee and a box of chocolate-covered macadamia nuts. I ate the chocolate, and put the coffee in the freezer. At the time, I didn't have a coffee brewer, and the present was never opened.

A few years later, I was offered a magazine story assignment that took me to Kauai. That was the first time I tasted Hawaiian. I was a guest at a woman's estate. I recall getting up early and drinking coffee and eating chocolate as we talked. The freshly brewed coffee paired with chocolates is a memory that I'll always cherish.

The third time around, I hit the Big Island. No work, just pleasure. Again, the coffee in the hotel room and at restaurants was not to be ignored. When I recall those days, I can close my eyes and taste the bold flavor of java. It's a tropical experience and one not to be forgotten.

Hawaiian coffee roasters will tell you that coffee is pricey because of the island's costly labor prices (it takes experts to pick beans). Kona is special and a challenge to get on the mainland. Sadly, these words make sense to me and perhaps that's one reason why trying to connect with a coffee company in Hawaii—and get a complimentary bag of beans—for this book was a challenge like riding a 50-foot swell.

But I did make an islands coffee connection. Meet David Gridley, president of Maui Oma Coffee Roasting Company. He answered my exclusive questions, one by one, telling me about the inside line of Hawaiian coffees—as difficult to get as gold, or so it seems.

"Most people come to us for our variety of Hawaiian coffees, mostly the Maui and Kona coffees," Gridley says, adding that they offer the Ka'u, Kauai, Molokai, and Waialua coffees as well.

Back in 1998 Gridley took the reins of the wholesale operation and Maui Oma was born, and it has ended up being a strong business to write home about. This means he supplies quality, fresh-roasted coffee (the Maui and Kona coffees are the most in demand) and sets up coffee programs for restaurants and coffee stores all over Hawaii and the mainland, my home.

I asked him, "Why is Hawaiian coffee considered so special?" He answered by telling me what I knew, but it was a sobering reminder: "Coffee is a tropical crop. It is really only grown between the Tropic of Cancer and the Tropic of Capricorn. This is why we are the only coffee-growing state. The best arabica coffees are grown at higher elevations, in volcanic soil, with sunny mornings and cloudy afternoons, and cool evenings."

So, he's in the right place. Perhaps that's why coffee in Hawaii costs more, and Gridley adds, "Yes, because the quality is high and demand is always higher than the availability. It also costs more to raise coffee in Hawaii. Land and labor costs are high." Meanwhile, as I fantasize moving to the Big Island, Gridley reminds me that there are many other emerging coffee-growing districts that are also growing some excellent and internationally recognized coffees.

Mexico: Though coffee in Mexico primarily comes from small coffee farms rather than large plantations, coffee farmers number over 100,000 and Mexico ranks as one of the largest coffee-producing countries in the world. A cup of Mexican coffee can offer a wonderful aroma and depth of flavor, often with a pronounced sharpness. It is an excellent bean for dark roasts and is often used in blends.

When I lived in the San Francisco Bay Area, a small authentic Mexican restaurant in San Carlos was my fave restaurant. After chips and salsa and a veggie lover's taco salad, I always ordered flan and a cup of Mexican coffee and it took me south of the border. Sweet Treat: Scones.

Puerto Rico: Coffees grown there are carefully cultivated from quality arabica varieties and produced to the highest standards. The coffees in this region are noted for their balanced body and acidity and fruity aroma. When I was a tween, one of my friends was from Puerto Rico. I recall after she visited her homeland she told me about sipping rum and coffee. Sweet Treat: Fresh fruit.

Central America

Guatemala: Guatemala's coffees have a distinctive taste quality favored by many for its flavor. A Guatemalan is a medium-to-full-bodied coffee, often with a depth and complexity of taste that is almost spicy on chocolaty to the tongue. Sweet Treat: Coffee chocolates. Guatemala Antigua (full City Roast coffee)—a fine coffee, it is rich, with a sweet and chocolaty flavor and a spicy, smooth, and long-lingering aftertaste, also boasting a bright, assertive acidity and full body. Sweet Treat: Chocolate bar.

Costa Rica: A Central American coffee-growing country with a reputation for its fine-quality coffee. It's touted for its medium body and sharp acidity—"perfect balance." Sweet Treat: Fresh berries or breakfast muffins.

South America

Colombia: Colombia, the world's best-known producer of coffee, ranks second worldwide in yearly production. Colombian Supremo, the highest grade, has a delicious, aromatic sweetness while Excelso Grade might be softer and slightly more acidic. Colombian coffee has made its way to my kitchen and Mr. Coffee. When I first tried it, I was clueless to its roots or flavor. Colombian is the coffee used for the flavored coffees that I discovered. Colombia (medium-roast coffee)— sweet aroma and flavor with overtones of caramel. It boasts a mild acidity, medium body, and is a wonderful breakfast coffee. Sweet Treat: Coffee cake (with fresh fruit).

Brazil: Brazil is the biggest coffee-producing country in the world. A "Brazilian" coffee is "mild" and the two terms are often used interchangeably. Brazilian is a clear, sweet, medium-bodied, low-acid coffee. Sweet Treat: Espresso bars or cookies. Brazil (dark-roast coffee)— Brazil Bobolink is from the dryer savanna-like Cerrado region; this semi-washed Brazil offers a deliciously smooth and soft cup. The dark-roast degree adds intensity to the medium-bodied, honey-nuanced flavor and spicy finish. Sweet Treat: Mocha brownies or tart.

Africa and the Middle East

East Africa

Ethiopia: Rewind to the place where coffee was discovered—a place where its people, like people around the world, enjoy this brew. Generally wet-processed, coffee from Ethiopia comes from one of three main growing regions—Sidamo, Harer, or Kaffa—and often bears one of those names. It is full flavored and a bit down-to-earth and full bodied. I was hesitant to try this dark coffee, assuming it wouldn't be as fun as the flavored coffees. I was wrong. Sweet Treat: Tiramisu.

Kenya: Kenyan coffee is well known and well liked in both the United States and Europe. Kenyan beans produce a singular cup of a sharp fruit acidity combined with full body and rich fragrance. Sweet Treat: Cheesecake.

West Africa

Ivory Coast: On the west coast of Africa, the Ivory Coast is one of the world's largest producers of robusta coffee. Coffees from the Ivory Coast are strongly aromatic, with a light body and acidity. They are ideal for a darker roast and are therefore often used in espresso blends. Sweet Treat: Chocolate coffee truffles.

The Arabian Peninsula

Yemen: In the country where coffee was first commercially cultivated one still finds coffee growing in the age-old century-proven manner. The Dutch combined Arabian coffee with coffee grown on the island of Java, thus making popular the first coffee blend—one that is still well known today—Mocha Java. Yemeni coffee has a distinctive taste that is deep, rich, and like no other. Sweet Treat: Mocha cake.

Asia

Civet Coffee, A Gourmet Treat

Let me introduce you to the Kopi Luwak bean gathered from the poop of civets (a small Asian Palm cat), which graze on coffee berries. It's the animals' droppings that are harvested by farmers who clean and ship the unchewed, undigested, and fermented commodity to people like Texas-based Dustin Butler, president of Bantai Civet Coffee (www.bantaicivetcoffee.com). Bantai's rare and pricey gourmet coffee (4 ounces cost $85; 16 ounces cost $320) comes from the Philippines (it is also found in Sumatra). After a bit of preliminary hesitation, I tasted the expensive and extremely smooth, almost buttery, coffee; it is not acidic like some coffees. Pure Civet Coffee is touted to taste both nutty and spicy. I'm still shocked that I braved brewing and sipping the rare coffee—but being a coffee and cat lover, how could I resist?

Indonesia: Today, small coffee farms of 1 or 2 acres predominate and most of the coffee is dry processed. Indonesian coffees are noted for a pronounced, rich, full body and mild acidity. Sweet Treat: Chocolate mousse.

Vietnam: Vietnam is rapidly becoming one of the world's largest coffee producers. Plantations located in the southern half of the country produce mostly robusta coffee. Vietnamese coffee has a light acidity and mild body with a good balance. It is frequently used for blending. Sweet Treat: Croissants.

(*Courtesy:* Data gleaned from the National Coffee Association of U.S.A, Inc. Some of these coffees are available at www.alpensierracoffee.com.)

Darling's Brew—A Dad's Sweet A.M.

As I stirred in the kitchen this morning grinding our daily brew, darling little Chloe, our three-year-old, asked, "Dad, let me smell the coffee" as she insists on being involved in making Mama's coffee whenever possible. The whir of the Virtuoso burr grinder filled the background as breaking sunlight filtered into the breakfast nook. "That smells good, Papa," Chloe says, with a big smile. I am confident that this little live wire is going to be a coffee achiever— sooner rather than later.

The Technivorm brewer begins its gurgle and the rays of morning light catch the ochre red of the first drops of brew in the pot. "Freeze this frame" is all I can think, as a soft and sweet moment occurs. No worries, a little darling by my side and the realization that the ochre red color of those first drops of brew is so rich that I am completely captivated. Wow, ochre red—the true color of the finest Arabica species coffee.

Then comes the aroma. With notes of rich cacao and spice, I look over and see that darling Chloe is anticipating the ensuing cup as much as I am. There is cause for excitement. The looming brew is capturing all of our senses and has us spellbound. What is it? It's one of our favorites, of course, and fresh from the farm. Guatemala Antigua Los Volcanes.

The Central American origin is just super, especially this time of year when the first bags have completed their "resting" phase and are arriving in port and in Minden to be expertly and skillfully brought to life by Alpen Sierra's production team. The acidity is so lovely and bright that it wakes the sense for a full blast of syrupy-sweet and rich chocolaty flavor. This comes from the double-washed processing the Guatemalans practice, which results in accentuated and clean acidity in the cup. As the rich mouth feel of this brew travels the palate, the finish becomes spicy and is long lingering in the aftertaste.[2]

SAVVY COFFEE-BREWING METHODS

The world of ways to brew a cup of coffee can be too complicated until you take the plunge and get to know the different methods. I'm still devoted to my auto drip Mr. Coffee—he's simple and works. (I still haven't programmed his automatic timer.) I almost had a fling with the French press, and the percolator takes me back to my days as a kid and adult during those camping times.

Each brewing tool has its flaws. Not one is perfect or for everyone. I think of coffee brewers as relationships. It's about how much you're willing to give to get results. Here, a glance at the basic Brew Tools—and what's in it for you.

1 **Filter Drip:** *Automatic Drip.* In an electric drip coffeemaker, like my Mr. Coffee, place the ground coffee in a paper liner fitted inside the machine's cone-shaped or round filter. Hot water is heated as it drips through the coffee bed, trickling into a pot that sits on the machine's warming plate or "burner."

   Pros. It's automatic and you can program the time anytime you want a quick and easy cup of coffee; it's complete with a simple cleanup.

   Cons. Eco-friendly folks may not race to power up for coffee, and the water is sometimes not as hot and steamy as other methods.

   The Manual Drip. A bit more high-maintenance than the automatic drip. Put ground coffee in the filter that is made to fit a filter holder that works with a carafe or mug. Heat the water, pour onto the coffee, and let it drip into your container.

   Pros. It's portion controlled, so waste not, want not; you control the coffee and water, and water temperature is hotter than the automatic drip.

   Cons. It's high maintenance, requiring more time and effort to boil water and pour the water through the coffee in the filter. Worse, if you're rushed, bits of coffee grounds may float in your cup of coffee.

2 **The Cold-Press:** Meet a larger white plastic container with its own filter. Fill the container with 1 pound of medium-ground coffee without stirring. Pour 4 cups of cold water over the coffee, wait 5 minutes, and repeat with 5 cups of water. Put in fridge

overnight to steep. The coffee liquid will drain through the filter into a carafe. Store the finished coffee in the sealed glass decanter and in the fridge till using.

Pros. Not only does it reduce acid, but it's also ideal for iced-coffee recipes.

Cons. The flavors of this method are not as high quality as the French press or espresso methods. A pound of coffee is a lot of coffee.

3 **The French Press:** Unlike the cold-press, this method had me ready to purchase one, but I didn't want to cope with buyer's remorse. It's a pot that is simple to work and promises a rich, steaming cup of java—without using electricity. Ground coffee infused with cooled, boiling water. Prewarm the glass beaker (rinse it with hot water). Put coffee in the beaker and fill with cool boiling water and put the lid on it. Steep for several minutes; then the plunger lid should be pressed down. This separates the finished coffee from the grounds, which are pressed to the bottom of the pot.

Pros. Tasty, less time consuming than drip methods, hot coffee, and it's portable like your companion animal—and budget wise at about $30.

Cons. The coffee may not be as hot once it's steeped; coffee grounds may stay on the bottom like a sick fish in an aquarium. What's more, unfiltered coffee may raise cholesterol.

4 **The Vacuum Pot:** If you're looking for a cup of excellent coffee, this method may be your last stop. Envision two glass globes, one set into another, with a filter, suspended over a heat source. (It looks like a kerosene lamp and can take you back in time if you have the time.) This method calls for a technical wizard. Fill the lower chamber with water and secure the upper chamber where you pour coffee grounds. Turn on your heat source—and wait. The water will heat and bubble. Take the pot off the heat and let the vacuum suck the liquid through the filter and back into the bottom carafe.

Pros. No sediment in your mug of coffee—it's pure and portable.

Cons. You may need Mr. Coffee (and a couple of cups of mud) to help you get through this ordeal—and some may feel the coffee is a bit too "thin."

5 **The Middle Eastern:** Meet a coffeepot aka an *ibrik*, or Turkish. Think of a long-handled metal pot with a wide base and narrow top. You can control the amount by putting in a couple of teaspoons of fine coffee with $1/2$ cup water. Boil. Once it foams, remove. Repeat. Let the grounds trickle to the bottom of your coffee mug before drinking.

Pros. A nice flavor and a rustic charm to this method.

Cons. Stray coffee grounds can be disturbing to finicky coffee drinkers. Sugar is often added, but added sugar isn't the healthiest route to take.

6 **The Percolator:** Last but not necessarily the least method to consider is boiling coffee like people did during the depression and in the forties. Fill the percolator with cold water. Place the ground coffee in the filter basket and insert the basket in the percolator. Cover and place on a lit stovetop burner or, if it is electric, plug it in, as my parents did in the fifties, and wait to hear the percolating sounds.

Pros. It's a nice old-fashioned way to brew coffee and takes you back to the slower-paced, low-tech world of *Father Knows Best*.

Cons. If you don't like a bitter cup of coffee or you cherish that steamy brew, this may not be your best bet. And note, like the French press, a hike in cholesterol may be linked to unfiltered coffee.

7 **Keurig K-Cup Home Brewer:** The words "K-Cup" continued to pop up during my research and I finally discovered what the mystery is. This brewing method is a single-serving brewing system. Coffee lovers purchase them for home use (and they are excellent for the workplace, too); they are available for both 6-ounce and 8-ounce cups.

Pros. In less than one minute you can have one cup of coffee, tea, or cocoa by using a K-Cup, which come in different coffee roasts; there's no waste if you're serving one.

Cons. The Keurig Home Brewer is more costly than other brewing methods.

8 **Coffee Pod Machines:** Like the Keuirg K-Cup Brewer, coffee pod machines are single-serve coffeemakers. Pods come in a single serving like a tea bag.

Pros. Less costly than a Keurig brewer. Coffee pod machines are offered in some hotels and guests are happy with the gourmet coffee pods. It's budget wise and ecofriendly. Did I mention you can enjoy a cup of coffee in less than one minute?

Cons. While this process is convenient for one person, if you have three or more people it can be too time consuming, taking more time than an automatic Mr. Coffee. Also, some pod brewers allow only for a 6-ounce cup, not ideal if you are used to drinking 12 ounces.

Me and Mr. Pod Brewer

During the dog days of summer, I had an affair with My Café: Single Serve Pod Brewer. It happened one afternoon when a large box from FedEx arrived on my doorstep. When I opened the brown box a coffee brewer box met my eyes. I was greeted with a handsome black and silver Bunn Café Pod Brewer. It was attraction at first sight, not one of those smaller types for college students. It was a good-looking brewer that had me once I took him out of the box. Several boxes of pods (Breakfast Blend, Colombian, French Roast, French Vanilla, Hazelnut, and Sumatra) came with the pod brewer, like a toy with extras that made me smile.

Like any new relationship, all was not perfect, because it was new and I didn't know what to expect. I'm not a techie. I admit that the manual intimidated me with its 11 step-by-step instructions. So, I plugged in the brewer. The Brew Button flashed red, a sign that it needed water and it was ready to set up. I had my favorite large 12-ounce white mug and put it on the Drip Tray under the Pod Drawer. Then, I opened the Spin Lid on top of my brewer and filled it with H_2O. The tricky part was when I pushed the Brew

Button—it's supposed to heat up the hot-water tank, but I wasn't sure it was the right way because the red button flashed.

I grabbed the manual and discovered he needed to be programmed to live with me in high altitude. So a few more tweaks and pushing the Pulse button five times—I was ready to place a French Vanilla pod in the pod drawer. I pressed the Brew Button, but only water dripped out. Oops, I didn't use enough water. So, I took out the first pod (it was wet) and inserted another one. I turned on the Brew Button and the green light was a sign all systems were a go. I heard the sound that it was going to run and yes, the coffee was dripping into my heat-resistant favorite large coffee cup.

Once done, I was amazed. No stray coffee grounds like with my Mr. Coffee machine. No messy filter and grounds. No leftover coffee. No cleanup. One large single serving of hot French Vanilla coffee was a done deal. Am I in love with my new brewer? Well, let's just say it's going to be a long, happy affair. Did I tell you how handsome he is? And yes, he is sitting on my kitchen countertop next to Mr. Coffee and my grinder. Thank you, Coffee.org, for hooking me up. I can use him for tea bags, too. I sense we're a match.

The Espresso Bar

Most of the coffee recipes and drinks that are popular at coffee shops and cafés today are based on espresso from the Old World. Espresso is not a coffee roast—it's the way coffee is made, by shooting hot water through ground coffee to produce an intense, flavorful beverage. An *Eat, Pray, Love* film image of an Italian espresso bar shows a crowded atmosphere with people standing and ordering their cappuccino or mocha from the barista, much like the more usual type of bar. Here is an espresso bar from A to Z:

Caffe Americano. This drink transforms espresso into more of an American brewed coffee. Start with one shot of espresso and add hot water to make a full 6-to-8-ounce cup. This results in a smooth, diluted version of espresso coffee.

Caffe Latte. Start with a single or double shot of espresso in a 10-to-12-ounce cup. Tilt the cup and pour about 8 to 10 ounces of steamed milk slowly down the side. This floats some of the espresso to the top, causing a swirling appearance. Sprinkle with nutmeg or cinnamon to garnish. As a common variation, latte can be flavored with Italian syrups such as hazelnut.

Caffe Mocha. This is made by adding powdered or chocolate syrup to a shot of espresso and blending. Add steamed milk to the espresso and chocolate mixture and top with whipped cream.

Cappuccino. This is made with one-third espresso, one-third steamed milk, and one-third frothed milk. Powdered cocoa or cinnamon can be sprinkled on the top as a garnish. To layer the milk and espresso, it's necessary to allow the frothed milk a moment to rest and separate.

Doppio. This is a double shot of espresso. "Doppio" means "double" in Italian. A double shot would be about twice that of a single shot, or 2 to 3 ounces of liquid.

Espresso con Panna. This is similar to macchiato, but whipped cream is used in place of the foamed milk. *Con panna* means "with cream" in Italian.

Espresso Macchiato. This starts with a shot of espresso and then a small amount of foamed milk is spooned over the shot. *Macchiato* means "marked" in Italian, referring to the espresso being marked with a spot of foam.

Espresso Romano. This is a single shot of expresso served with a twist of lemon peel. Contrary to the name Romano, this is not an Italian tradition. The lemon-peel garnish is actually a U.S. invention.

Mochaccino. This is similar to caffe mocha, but topped with peaked milk foam instead of whipped cream.

Ristretto. This is the short or ristretto and is a basic espresso shot extracted to a volume of only ¾ ounce of liquid. This restricted pour magnifies the essence and intensity even more than a normal espresso being marked with a spot of foam.

Straight Shot. This is a single straight shot of espresso, without any other ingredients, about 1 to 1.5 ounces of liquid. Espresso, when made right, will have a rich layer of golden crema on the top. . . . Be sure to drink the espresso right away—the crema will only last about 2 minutes and then it will dissolve into the liquid.

(*Courtesy:* Gourmet Coffee Zone.)

Now that I've infused coffee roasts from around the globe into your brain and methods to brew the java of your choice, in the next chapter you'll discover the wide world of flavored coffees. Every morning I wake up to making a decision: "What flavor of coffee should I brew?" Blueberry crumble, pumpkin spice, chocolate raspberry, and Irish cream—these are just four of dozens of flavors I tried and vowed to keep in my kitchen year round.

A CUP FULL OF PERKS

✓ There is an art to tasting coffee—the good and the bad of its flavor and layers of acidity, body, characteristics, and roast tastes.
✓ Coffees are derived from around the world, including Hawaii, Mexico, South America, and other regions—all with their own special merits.
✓ Brewing methods are varied and each one has its upside and downside, including health benefits and convenience factors.
✓ Espresso is not a type of coffee; it's a type of brewing method and used for an intense base coffee in many espresso drinks, from cappuccino to lattes.

Flavored Coffees

During my junior college days in San Jose, California, I scheduled
back-to-back classes that demanded the help of hot liquid energy
(black coffee in a thermos). I endured the commute because I was
alert and studied en route on the train and bus (think a female version
of Abraham Lincoln going the extra mile to get an education). But my
school days during this chapter of my undergraduate life were grueling
because I had to work, too—and comforting flavored coffee came to
the rescue.

Once I got home I tended to Mildred, an elderly widow cooped up
like a bird in her blue and white upscale trailer. A typical night went
like this: As I sipped a cup of flavored coffee (the store bought instant
kind) I fixed dinner for her and chow for her Pomeranian and my black
Labrador, Stone Fox. After the dog walks, I gave the widow a perm. I
listened to her detailed stories about her late husband, estranged kids,
and grandchildren. The widow, who fought a bad hip and brittle-bone
disease, was in pain and alone—except for me, her confidante. It was

the caffeine fix that helped me to get through this second shift of my school days.

After my chores, "Millie" let me use her bathroom spa. I drew a hot bubble bath and clicked on the Jacuzzi switch. The best part was a fresh cup of steamy vanilla coffee. It was a decadent delight that took me back in time to when my grandmother let me drink Coke and eat marshmallow cookies in the bathtub like the Romans who used to enjoy the natural mineral springs in the village of Spa in Belgium.

As time passed, so did Mildred's dog. Three months later, the woman did not make it through an operation for her hip. I moved on, but my sweet coffee nights are a memory that I will always cherish.

THE HISTORY OF FLAVORED JAVA...

Enter the wide world of flavored coffees, which is as old as the as the beverage itself—much like hot chocolate. Adding flavors, such as cardamom and mint leaf, goes back to coffee's earliest days in the Middle East. The addition of sugar and milk as flavor additives goes back hundreds of years in the West, explains New York–based Gillies Coffee Company's founder Donald Schoenholt. He adds that flavored coffees were a growing trend in the early 1980s—the same time I turned to those gourmet store–bought instant beverages.

Some companies that introduced flavored coffees include Maxwell House, whose International Instant Coffees used powdered milk as an ingredient, and independent specialty roasters such as Gillies, which use flavored coffee beans. Also, Van Cortland Coffee in Moonachie, New Jersey, Superior Coffee & Tea Company in Chicago, Illinois, and First Colony Coffee & Tea Company in Norfolk, Virginia, played a part in the flavored coffee parade that has blossomed into the 21st century.

THE SECRETS OF FLAVORED COFFEES

These days, flavored coffees (available in the form of beans and ground) are found and favored at gourmet coffee shops, grocery stores, online specialty coffee roasters, and retailers. "Flavored coffees are often made by adding flavoring liquid to roast coffee beans, or adding a dry flavoring compound to ground coffee," says Schoenholt. "There are flavored coffees manufactured with all natural ingredients. These are flavored with vanilla bean, cinnamon, and other easily added natural substances."

It is noteworthy, adds the coffee wizard, that all-natural ingredients have some disadvantages. For one, they can be costly because they are subject to allergen labeling to the fact that natural ingredients may cause the flavored coffee to spoil.

I did jump on the Starbucks flavored-coffee bandwagon before I tackled *The Healing Powers of Coffee* and discovered different flavors, thanks to our friendly Safeway. Before my assignment, I rotated Cinnamon and Vanilla Hazelnut—these two flavored coffees were my first experience with flavored coffee beans. I often bought a bag of the ground coffee. But my flavored-coffee experiences expanded.

Coffee, Tea & Spice, based in Oklahoma, is a newer company that I found online and introduced me to a new world of flavored coffees. They opened their online business in 2005. Flavored coffees make up about 40 percent of all of their sales; their most popular flavors are Snickerly-Cookie, White Chocolate Mousse, and Highlander Grogg. The flavored coffees are not natural flavors because too many people suffer from allergies—so they turn to artificial flavors for their Colombian Supremo coffee beans (other coffee companies turn to Colombian for flavored concoctions, too). Chocolate- and fruit-flavored coffees also rank high with their customers. Owner Mary adds, "Coffee and chocolate have a trigger for the senses that makes you feel calm, relaxed, and it does something for you that no other food does." As one who has a keen sense of smell, I agree.

THE COFFEE FLAVOR PARADE

Here, take a look at popular coffee flavors, 25 that I've tasted and enjoyed, and I would love to go for another 25 and probably will do just that. There are hundreds of flavored coffees to choose from. These days, like centuries ago, mixing these coffees with dark chocolate, spices, and citrus can make them more flavorful.

The aroma of flavored coffee can be chocolaty, fruity, nutty, minty, and spicy. And personally, I treasure seasonal flavored coffees, such as pumpkin spice—it reminds me of eating autumn delights, including pumpkin fudge, ice cream, muffins, and pie. I adore German chocolate cake and southern pecan, too. Each different flavor is distinct, much like trying a different chocolate or honey flavor. But there are so many other flavors that can please the palate, too.

BLUEBERRY CRUMBLE: I love fresh blueberries. These gems can often be found in blueberry scones, muffins, pound cake, and corn-bread—and now flavored coffee. So, when I opened this coffee bag and read the description "The essence of a Blueberry Cinnamon Crumb cake" I thought, "Yes! I've baked a blueberry coffee cake." Think blueberry treats, like these, with a touch of spice. *Best Blends:* Team with pancakes or waffles, fruit scones, or cinnamon toast. *My Personal Tasting:* I savored a cup of this flavored berry coffee with a bowl of hot oatmeal and fresh blueberries to celebrate the summer-time fruit that can be pricey off season. This combination makes it a challenge to go back to strong black coffee without an extra kick of berries year-round.

BRAZILIAN SUNSET: At first, this flavor didn't do anything to my imagination, but the descriptive words "A fantasy flavor—naturally nutty with overtones of coconut" promised an exotic coffee that cap-tivated me. *Best Blends:* Chocolate biscotti, cake, or cookies work like a charm. *My Personal Tasting:* I took out the dark chocolate biscotti, dipped into this flavorful, rich coffee, and discovered each dunk was worth the effort. I like sunrises, but this coffee took me back in time to a Florida Keys sunset that I once enjoyed and Floridians can enjoy every day. A cup of this flavored Brazilian coffee would do any sunset anywhere justice.

BUTTERSCOTCH TOFFEE: Speaking of beautiful sunsets, the sweet buttery taste of butterscotch on sundaes and in candy as a kid is still with my memories as an adult. Butterscotch and Colombian cof-fee are like two perfect tastes with my name on it. *Best Blends:* A bagel, croissant, or slice of pound cake is perfect with a cup of this double duo of sweetened coffee without the calories of rich desserts. *My Personal Tasting:* The taste reminded me of a gourmet coffee with those flavored syrups. But the coffee was just as good without extras, including creamers and whipped cream.

CHERRY VANILLA CRÈME: Cherries like blueberries are rich in antioxidants. While the flavorings do not contain the same compounds as the fruit, you are getting a dose of good-for-you coffee that tastes like cherries and cream. How sweet is that? So, it's up to you to power up the coffee with foods. The description on the bag of Cherry Vanilla Crème read: "Tangy cherry blended with smooth vanilla crème." *Best Blends:* Anything dark chocolate (such as ice cream and truffles) is a super mate with cherry vanilla crème coffee. *My Personal Tasting:* A square of 70 percent cacao content chocolate bar with a steamy cup of this cherry delight—a bit thin and not full bodied like Hawaiian Hazelnut—I topped it with a dollop of whipped cream and a dash of cocoa powder. This creamy cherry coffee triggered a knockoff of Black Forest cake—without the fat and calories.

CHOCOLATE HAZELNUT: Real superfoods, including cherries, chocolate, and nuts, all boast antioxidants, but that's not the only reason why I love them. The idea of pairing the two makes sense and gives the promise of a double delight. Chocolaty coffees and nut coffees are in demand, coffee retailers and roasters tell me. *Best Blends:* Pair with plain cheesecake to cheeses and fresh fruit. *My Personal Tasting:* I brewed a cup of this chocolate lover's coffee and teamed it with gourmet ginger biscotti. Getting the overlapping flavors of chocolate, hazelnut, and ginger was a fine mix and the crunchy Italian cookie made it work on all levels.

CHOCOLATE RASPBERRY: Another chocolate-flavored coffee caught my eye. I sent one bag of this coffee to my webmaster. I regretted doing that, especially when she told me how she loved the hints of both chocolate and fruit flavors. Karma paid me a visit and another bag of this coffee ended up on my doorstep. And yes, she was right. *Best Blends:* Chocolate with chocolate is deliciousness, including dark chocolate bars, dark chocolate truffles, and dark chocolate ice cream. *My Personal Tasting:* I enjoyed a small scoop each of all-natural premium French vanilla ice cream and drizzled a cup of hot chocolate raspberry coffee on top. It gave this coffee treat a Mediterranean flair. One summer afternoon, I treated myself to a small fresh-brewed cup of chocolate raspberry coffee after a homemade egg salad sandwich with lots of spring greens and tomatoes on a whole-grain roll. No ice cream needed.

CINNAMON: The first time I tried this treat was via Starbucks—a bag of beans that I purchased at Safeway—and before I entered Coffee

World. Since then, specialty roasters and retailers have sent me bags of this flavor and they tell me it's one of the most popular. *Best Blends:* This versatile and well-loved flavored coffee goes with breakfast foods, whether it is eggs and toast or a bowl of whole-grain cereal, hot or cold. Also, it's ideal for dessert after dinner. *My Personal Tasting:* I adore cinnamon coffee with a bagel or homemade scone topped with cream cheese and fresh strawberries. It also gives a creamy egg custard with a dash of nutmeg a spicy twist throughout all four seasons.

CINNAMON HAZELNUT: If you like sweet cinnamon-flavored coffee, you may love cinnamon hazelnut brew. Cinnamon goes back centuries to flavor tea, cakes, and cookies. *Best Blends:* Breads, muffins, cakes, and pies are good mates with notes of cinnamon and hazelnut. *My Personal Tasting:* Sitting on the deck underneath the pine trees and feeling the warm sunshine, I peeled a pricey summertime orange one morning. After, I sipped a fresh-brewed cup of this coffee and it whisked me away to a bistro abroad. Simple flavors like cinnamon and hazelnut sometimes are better than complex ones. An extra bonus: The aroma of cinnamon hazelnut coffee lingering through the kitchen, dining room, and on the deck is like baking cinnamon cookies or rolls without the work.

COCONUT CRÈME: During the summertime and sometimes during the winter I crave getting on a jet plane and visiting the Hawaiian Islands. A taste of the islands—coconut crème flavored coffee—boasts a smooth coffee with a subtle coconut flavor. *Best Blends:* This tropical java is ideal with fresh fruit, including pineapple, strawberries, and kiwi fruit. Dark chocolate and milk chocolates pair well, too. *My Personal Tasting:* I've mastered the art of making rice pudding. Warm or refrigerated, this creamy, wholesome pudding made with whole-grain rice is perfect with a cup of iced coconut crème coffee in the summer and hot when the temperatures plummet. It's a year-round treat.

DANISH PASTRY: The aroma of coconut crème coffee is exotic, but this Danish pastry flavored coffee is oh-so sweet, like those day-old Danishes I'd purchase in San Francisco on the way home from college classes. No need to grab a gooey Danish pastry with unwanted sugar, calories, and fat. *Best Blends:* Fresh fruit and tossed green salads are good for you with this sweet coffee as dessert. *My Personal Tasting:* This coffee was fun and pairing it with berries, peaches, to a fresh apple was sublime. The best part is, I felt like I was getting a pastry, but instead I was getting Colombian coffee and a sweet fix in a healthier way. This is one flavored coffee to put on my list of favorite fun flavored coffees— and one for colder days, colder nights, and the first snowfall.

DARK CHOCOLATE MINT: Chocolaty coffees are popular and for good reason. Both chocolate and coffee go back centuries. The pairing works and it works for me. The dark chocolate mint beans woke me up with the aroma—a hint that I'd be satisfied with the first sip one morning. *Best Blends:* Butter cookies and chocolate cheesecake put this coffee in its sweet place. *My Personal Tasting:* I enjoyed this flavored coffee solo before breakfast. As simple as it sounds, teaming Mother Nature's sweetest summertime fruits with dark chocolate mint coffee creates a treat that is memorable, light, and fat burning, if you're watching your weight or want to keep your weight in check.

ETHIOPIAN HARRAR: Unlike the dark chocolate mint flavored beans that I liked for the flavor and scent, this fruit-like, spice specialty coffee bag wasn't noticed. As I researched flavors of coffee it kept coming up, so I saw that as a sign to give it a try. *Best Blends:* A mix of flavors makes a coffee like this go well solo or with fruit, muffins, and bagels. *My Personal Tasting:* On a summer morning I made a batch of bran pineapple muffins. Instead of grabbing a bag of a chocolaty coffee, I decided it was time to try this one with a warm muffin. To my surprise this flavor was smooth and better than other familiar-type flavored coffees.

FRENCH CARAMEL: Like chocolate, I love caramel. *Best Blends:* Bagel with cream cheese, plain croissants, butter cookies, chocolate biscotti, chocolate cake, and custard go perfectly with this addictive coffee flavor. *My Personal Tasting:* Before I began writing *The Healing Powers of Coffee*, I was hooked on Starbucks French Caramel coffee. (I've also dropped a caramel or used caramel syrup in java coffee, which is heavenly for coffee and caramel lovers.) Every morning when I'd brew a cup of French caramel, a splash of milk was enough to give me a perfect sweet taste without flavorings: sugar, cream, or whipped cream.

FRENCH VANILLA: Like French caramel flavored coffee, French vanilla had me at its title and description on the bag of beans: "A flavored coffee favorite! Smooth vanilla notes embrace a rich Colombian coffee." Oh, the aroma of the beans is wonderful. *Best Blends:* Fruit, yogurt, pastries. *My Personal Tasting:* I enjoyed this coffee flavor on more than one occasion. I recall the morning I made a healthful Orange Julius. I sipped this coffee (the scent permeating my kitchen) while I juiced oranges and fed my trusty blender with fresh OJ, a few scoops of premium French vanilla ice cream, low-fat organic milk, 1 tablespoon orange blossom honey, a few tablespoons of confectioner's sugar, 1/4 teaspoon pure vanilla extract, and ice cubes. I was in vanilla heaven and the French vanilla coffee took me there.

GERMAN CHOCOLATE CAKE: The aroma of this chocolaty coffee is memorable. While the title (from Oh! Nuts) is sublime, I wasn't sure if the taste would match the images of this dessert with sweet chocolate, nuts, and coconut. *Best Blends:* Paired with premium chocolate or vanilla ice cream or fresh berries is a good choice. *My Personal Tasting:* I sipped this flavored coffee with a plain but healthful breakfast. The chocolaty flavor with notes of nuts and coconut took me to a place that is for java junkies. I was hooked. Note to self: Order this unforgettable chocolate-coffee lovers' flavored coffee.

HAWAIIAN HAZELNUT: While the German chocolate cake was a coffee that made me smile, I wasn't sure the same would happen with the flavored islands one with hazelnut. Because it came from the Alpen Sierra Coffee Roasting Company, I sensed it would be a high-quality coffee—but perhaps not fun. *Best Blends:* Ideal with eggs and hash browns or chocolate-chip pancakes. *My Personal Tasting:* This flavored coffee moved fast in my household. Its rich and smooth flavor won my taste buds, and it was one beverage I served to family and friends. It's a coffee that you'll want to show off because it's not a girlie flavored coffee—it's real and it's one that people will request a second cup, not small size, either.

HIGHLANDER GROGG COFFEE: This flavored coffee is touted as a "rich, full flavor, similar to Drambuie"—and I admit that this wasn't my first choice, but it is favored by flavored-coffee drinkers, so it aroused my curiosity. I am not a drinker of alcohol; I took to this non-alcoholic coffee noted for its taste of Scottish brandy with a butter and spice flavor. I used more beans than less for a stronger flavor and its aroma panned out to a pleasurable brew. *Best Blends:* Nice with whole-grain crackers, mild cheddar cheese, and fruit. Or a premium ice cream. *My Personal Tasting:* I paired this flavored coffee with a slice of cheesecake drizzled with honey. It was a decadent treat.

IRISH CREAM: *Best Blends:* Eggs, scones, and toast are fine with this old-fashioned favorite flavored coffee. *My Personal Tasting:* From time to time, I will make a hearty Irish breakfast: scrambled eggs, toast, fried potatoes—and this Irish cream coffee with milk and a dollop of whipped cream completed the meal. Like other flavored coffees, this one has its place, whether it is with a special breakfast or in the afternoon sitting by a crackling fire during a snowy day. Its refreshing aroma is captivating and once you taste this flavored coffee more than likely you'll want to taste it again. It would be perfect for a fall afternoon after a walk or swim or on a cold, wintry night during the first snowfall.

MAPLE PECAN: Like chocolate, I adore syrup, the pricey, pure kind. It's worth it. So this flavor of coffee, like drizzles of maple syrup on toasted pecans, caught my coffee lover's eye with a promise to titillate my taste buds. *Best Blends:* This sweet, nutty coffee is made for sipping with a bowl of oatmeal or a hot croissant with real butter. *My Personal Tasting:* Scrambled eggs, a toasted whole-grain bagel, and a cup of maple pecan flavored coffee were a breakfast that I'll cherish. It was a summery morning—quiet and cool with a promise of a warm day. I sat outside on the deck amid blue jays and under the towering pine trees, but the taste of pecan took me away to a great escape that could have been many places with a serene environment.

PUMPKIN SPICE: The sweet taste of pumpkin is a fall classic. Pumpkin spice boasts an array of cloves and spices, including cinnamon and ginger. That means this coffee drink is good for digestive woes, heart health, and as an anti-inflammatory. *Best Blends:* Pair pumpkin spice coffee with French toast, soups, and for a double punch a slice of pumpkin pie with a dollop of whipped cream. *My Personal Tasting:* My first experience with this flavored coffee was at Starbucks. It was at a hotel resort after a prewinter morning swim. I confess that I adore anything pumpkin and I knew that I'd love this flavored coffee prepared in the comfort of my cabin. It brought me back to that cold, romantic outdoor swim, exciting gambling splurge, and hot coffee prepared for me. I topped the beverage with a dash of nutmeg (another favorite) and was in coffee heaven. What's more, I don't have to wait until October to enjoy this warm cup of flavored coffee.

Roastin' Holiday Flavored Coffees

Welcome to Jelks premium coffee, which was established in 1896. Between 1976 and 1980, Jelks Gourmet Coffee Roasters, in Shreveport, Louisiana, saw the demand for flavored coffee and began with about five flavors. Since then, Jelks has added a few flavors every year. They roast more than 200 flavors.

One thing that makes their coffee stand out is that they use a gourmet blend of coffees (instead of single origin) to produce their flavored coffee. What's more, Jelks uses 100 percent arabica coffee, heat sealed in a 12-ounce bag, with a one-way valve to keep the coffee fresh. And they claim their flavored coffee has no calories, sugar, carbs, and cholesterol. They do use both natural and artificial flavors.

I can personally attest that their wide assortment of holiday flavored coffees (including Egg Nog Crème Brûlée, Gingerbread, Mistletoe Delight, and Thanksgiving Blend) wowed me with the flavors, aroma, and taste. Every morning during November and December, I felt the holiday spirit when I savored a special flavor of my choice for the morning or afternoon.

Choosing specialty flavored coffees for the festive fall/holiday season is worth the extra time and effort. Online I discovered other coffee roasters (www.gourmetcoffee express.com), who also made my holidays sweet. It was the Cinnamon Sweet Potato Swirl and Sugar & Spice Cake that were unforgettable to me.

SOUTHERN PECAN: Here is a mellow, slightly nutty flavored coffee that is one that I tried sooner rather than later. I adore nutty coffees and nuts. So, I sensed this coffee would be a good prospect. *Best Blends:* Muffins, oatmeal, and fresh fruit all are great pairings for this nutty coffee. *My Personal Tasting:* I'm not one for supersweet breakfasts (except sometimes blueberry waffles or chocolate-chip pancakes can tempt me). So, with southern pecan I teamed it with fresh fruit (bananas, raspberries, and strawberries), and whole grain toast. It was the coffee that made a simple breakfast a sweet treat.

SNICKERLY-COOKIE: I was definitely interested in trying this coffee, noted as the most popular flavored coffee, named after a cookie. The descriptive phrase "a delicious blend of cinnamon, hazelnut, and vanilla—just like the cookie!" is enough to snag anyone's interest who likes these flavors and remember these cookies. *Best Blends:* Plain cereal, fresh fruit, or as an after-dinner dessert beverage works well. *My Personal Tasting:* The aroma wowed me and the taste is one that left me thinking: "I wish I had more." This coffee is one of the most popular flavored coffees and I can see why. It's special with its special blend of special spices that are favored by me and countless others around the world. Its cutesy name delivers a taste that I take seriously.

SUGAR PLUM PUDDING: A blast from the past with sugar cookies is one thing, but indulging in a coffee that brings back memories of an English holiday classic with its blend of nutmeg, cinnamon, raisins, and a splash of brandy may take you back in time to the 17th century. *Best Blends:* This coffee is so amazing that it's the best solo to be savored for all of its special flavors. *My Personal Tasting:* On a day when I was feeling like a cold was paying me a visit (thanks to too-early A.M. dog walks and late work nights), I treated myself to this special flavored coffee. I craved nurturing, which a cup of coffee can do. Underneath the comforters, with the view of pine trees to the left and right of me from the windows in my bedroom, flanked by my two cuddly Brittanys and cat, Zen—sipping a cup of this flavored coffee comforted me. The sweet, spicy flavor made me feel better despite my throat being sore.

TIRAMISU: Imagine a coffee that tastes silky, smooth, and similar to the Italian dessert capturing ladyfingers, mascarpone cheese, vanilla, espresso, chocolate, rum, and cocoa powder. *Best Blends:* A cup of this European-type coffee can be paired with biscotti, bagels, a Bundt cake, or fresh fruit, such as green and purple grapes. *My Personal Tasting:* This is one flavored coffee that grabbed my interest and my first sip was full of sensory detail, from aroma to the rich, smooth taste. I dipped gourmet almond biscotti (which I had frosted with a home-made dark chocolate frosting) into the hot cup of sweet coffee and it was a sensory delight. This coffee paired with the Italian cookie was such a special team that I'll definitely serve it again (solo) and to friends and family.

WILD BLACKBERRY: Tiramisu is awesomeness, but a wild black-berry coffee is a fantasy coffee, too. Imagine fresh blackberries and pair them with a rich Colombian coffee and you get the West Coast and South America. *Best Blends:* This flavored coffee is perfect with a custard pudding or pie, plain toast or bagels, and a rich chocolate cake or cupcakes. *My Personal Tasting:* I brewed a cup of wild blackberry and served up a slice of New York cheesecake topped with fresh black-berries. No, it wasn't overkill with blackberries, it was blackberry heaven.

(These flavored coffees were provided to me by Gilles Coffee; Coffee, Tea & Spice; White Coffee Company; Coffee.org. Quotation descriptions gleaned from Coffee, Tea & Spice.)

Life Goes On with Cappuccino Bliss

On Sunday, May 22, after being dog-tired from following the May 21 end of the world prediction (and my anti-prediction on national radio and in print media), I turned to prepackaged gourmet biscotti and a cappuccino mix. I glanced at the coffeepot, which still had fresh-brewed cof-fee in it. I gave the crispy confections (with nuts) a java frosting spread and paired it with the beverage. Sure, it wasn't made by a sophisticated barista at an espresso bar, but it was toffee flavored and easy to make.

Sweet Cappuccino

In a small saucepan, put ½ cup of water; in another saucepan put ½ cup of 2 percent organic low-fat milk. At the same time, boil water and heat milk, but do not boil. Remove from stovetop. Put 2 to 3 teaspoons of instant flavored cappuccino mix into an 8-ounce coffee cup. Pour in milk and water. Stir well. Add a dollop of whipped cream and mix till frothy. Sprinkle with a dash of cinnamon. Serves 1.

COFFEE'S CONSTANT COMPANIONS: NATURAL SPICES

A feature on the Oldways Mediterranean Diet Pyramid is spices, for reasons of both health and taste. Also, spices contribute to the natural identities of various Mediterranean cuisines. Here are a few of my favorite herbs and spices to team with different regular coffees—not the flavored types.

Cardamom (Elettaria cardamomum): Here is a special coffee pairing treat often used in Egypt paired with coffee, past and present. It's a healing herb that may help soothe tummy troubles. It goes well with chocolaty coffees.

Cinnamon (Cinnamomum zeylanicum): The delicious taste of hot cinnamon buns with sticky honey and the warm memories they invoke in me from childhood when I smelled a homemade apple pie baking in the oven. The earthy, inviting flavor of cinnamon has been used worldwide by a multitude of cultures for its versatile seasoning powers as well as for its healing powers for thousands of years.

Cinnamon comes from the bark of the cinnamon tree found mostly in Ceylon and China. It can be found in several forms, including the stick, which can be grated or used to stir or season beverages—such as hot chocolate and apple cider. In ground form, it is the most common spice used for seasoning and baking. There are countless flavored coffees that include cinnamon, one of nature's finest spices that spice up java well and also provide medicinal properties. It is used in chocolaty coffees.

Mint (Menthapipertita and Menthaviridis): Both peppermint and mint can soothe tension and help you to relax, but mint can also calm a queasy stomach. It's a great addition to coffee after a meal or decaf before bed. Or a cup of hot chocolate with plenty of warm milk and mint can help you have sweet dreams.

Vanilla (Vanilla): Vanilla-flavored coffees are popular, like cinnamon-flavored ones. In folklore, it was believed vanilla boasts aphrodisiac perks for both men and women. The scent of vanilla-flavored coffee can be arousing and the taste can also titillate the palate whether you're a couple or solo.

Chocolate-Mocha Flan

❖ ❖ ❖

1½ ounces finely chopped bittersweet chocolate
2½ cups 1 percent low-fat milk
5 tablespoons pure maple syrup
1½ teaspoons ground cinnamon
2 teaspoons instant coffee or espresso granules

2 eggs
3 egg whites
2 teaspoons Kahlúa or coffee brandy
Confectioners' sugar for garnish
Fresh mint sprigs for garnish

Preheat the oven to 350°F. Combine the chocolate, milk, and maple syrup in a saucepan set over medium-low heat. Bring to a simmer, stirring constantly, until the chocolate has melted. Be careful not to boil the milk or it may scorch, giving the flan a burned bitter flavor. Remove from the heat and stir in the cinnamon and instant coffee. Set aside and let cool slightly.

Whisk the eggs, egg whites, and Kahlúa or coffee brandy in a mixing bowl. Slowly pour the warm milk mixture into the egg mixture in a thin stream, whisking constantly so the eggs do not scramble. Strain through a fine-mesh sieve to remove any milk solids and any remaining foam. (This is also the way to save the dish if the eggs start to scramble.)

Pour equal amounts of flan batter into 10 ramekins and

place them into a large, deep pan. Fill the pan with enough water to come one-third of the way up the sides of the ramekins. Be careful not to get any water into the ramekins. Bake for 45 minutes to 1 hour or until the flan is firm. Remove from the oven and let cool to room temperature. Garnish with confectioners' sugar and mint sprigs.

(Reprinted with permission from *The Golden Door Cooks Light & Easy,* by Chef Michel Stroot, published by Gibbs Smith, 2003.)

In the next chapter, "Sweet Mates," you'll find out that coffee is complemented and healthified with milk—all types—and sabotaged with sugar, cream, and artificial sweeteners. Also, coffee is found in foods, from candy and ice cream to yogurt and chocolate. The best part is, these combinations are often good for you, thanks to healing coffee and its powers.

A Cup Full of Perks

✓ Popular flavored coffees are French Vanilla and Hazelnut.
✓ Flavored coffees can be categorized in groups, including chocolaty, fruity, mint, and spice . . .
✓ . . . And seasonal flavored coffees offer a wide range, from pumpkin spice and sugar plum pudding to chocolate raspberry and coconut cream.
✓ Colombian coffee is often the choice of coffee used for flavored coffees.
✓ Both natural and artificial ingredients are used to flavor the coffees due to a variety of reasons, from cost-effectiveness to consumers' health reasons, such as allergies.
✓ Flavored coffees have been popular for years, and these days their popularity has soared to both commercial and specialty gourmet brands.
✓ To keep flavored coffees healthy, stay clear of adding sugar and syrups. Instead, enjoy them as is or with milk.
✓ Ready-made flavored coffees are convenient and irresistible, but adding your own natural flavors, whether it is cinnamon sticks or dark chocolate shavings, offers a fresh flair and healthful touch.

PART 4

MORE COFFEE COMPANIONS

Sweet Mates

A certain Liquor which they call Coffee . . . which
will soon intoxicate the brain.
—G. W. Parry (1601)[1]

After my ready-made flavored instant coffee period, I regressed to regular coffee but had a thing for adding milk. Flavored coffees weren't in
my starving student life on a shoestring budget. I was hooked, though,
on coffee nips (inexpensive hard candies) that I bought in the school
bookstore.

One midterm week on a Monday, I ditched classes (like my hooky
coffee days back in grade school) and bought a large cup of rocket fuel
(strong coffee) at the San Francisco State University Student Union. I
studied for tests and watched soap operas—a three-hour coffee soap-
athon. I was hooked—soaps and coffee. Once the caffeine jolt worked
its magic, it was tempting to put my creativity to work and fine-tune
my story about traveling through the desert with a talking box for a
creative writing workshop instead of tackling $Y + Z$ problems for a
math class exam.

The next afternoon I studied at home in the Santa Cruz Mountains. My yellow Labrador, Carmella, was pregnant and her pups were
due any hour. Like a dedicated midwife I stayed up with my loyal girl

and drank instant coffee with hot milk instead of boiling water (like people in Spain and India do) to keep alert and calm. The first pup was a challenge. It wasn't breathing. At midnight, I called the ER vet and they talked me through the life-or-death ordeal. Eleven pups later, we were all whupped. The cups of jolt got me through the night and days that followed. Thanks to the daily infusion, I got through a backyard breeder's job, from tuning out weaning cries 24/7 to cleaning up constant puppy mega spills. I believed there was a God who loves both dogs and coffee.

MILK IN YOUR COFFEE?

Black coffee is good for you; black coffee with milk is better. Personally, I prefer organic regular low-fat milk. I recall, however, the days of Tahoe winters when my coffee-drinking habit was equal parts of organic chocolate low-fat milk—like Germans and Swiss drink.

Cow's milk is chock full of nutrients that help support your body from head to toe. It is an excellent source of protein, calcium, and phosphorus. Many dairy foods are fortified with vitamins A and D, which are essential for human health, including building stronger bones. Here, straight from the people who know milk, are some facts that will help you decode different types of the white stuff you've been putting in your cup of coffee.

Types of Milk

There are many types of cow's milk available on the market today to meet a wide range of consumer preferences and health concerns. The primary types of milk sold in stores are: whole milk, reduced-fat milk (2 percent), low-fat milk (1 percent), and fat-free milk. The percentages included in the names of the milk indicate how much fat is in the milk by weight; whole milk contains 3.5 percent milk fat, reduced-fat milk contains at least 2 percent milk fat, and low-fat contains 1 percent milk fat. Fat-free, also called nonfat or skim, milk contains no more than 0.2 percent milk fat. Reduced-fat milks contain all of the nutrients found in whole milk.

Organic milk is produced by dairy farmers who use only organic fertilizers and organic pesticides, and their cows are not given supplemental hormones. Organic milk is also available as lactose free and ultra-pasteurized. The nutrient content of organic milk is the same as standard milk and organic milk offers no additional health benefits compared to standard milk.

Pasteurization requires heating the milk to destroy harmful microorganisms and prolong shelf life. Normal pasteurization keeps milk safer while maintaining valuable nutrients. After pasteurization, milk undergoes homogenization to prevent separation of the milk from the fluid milk. Finally, milk is fortified to increase its nutritional value or to replace nutrients lost during processing. Vitamin D is added to most milk produced in the United States to facilitate the absorption of calcium.

Raw milk has not been pasteurized. Proponents of drinking raw milk often claim that raw milk is more nutritious than pasteurized milk and that raw milk is inherently antimicrobial, thus making pasteurization unnecessary. In fact, raw milk spoils significantly faster than pasteurized milk, further increasing the risk of harmful bacteria spreading, causing illness. Raw milk, no matter how carefully produced, can contain unhealthful bacteria and microorganisms such as salmonella, *E. coli,* and listeria. The Centers for Disease Control and the Food and Drug Administration firmly support the use of pasteurized milk and milk products, cautioning consumers that the harmful bacteria in raw milk may cause life-threatening illnesses.

Lactose-free milk is available for individuals who are unable to break down lactose, the natural sugar found in milk. Lactose-free milk is a convenient way for lactose-intolerant individuals to consume milk and its beneficial nutrients.

(Adapted from information from The California Dairy Council.)

MILK NUTRIENTS

MILK (1 CUP)—FEDERAL STANDARDS

	Fat-free	Low-fat 1%	Reduced-fat 2%	Whole	Chocolate 1%
Calories	90	101	122	152	158
Protein (g)	8	8	8	8	8
Carbohydrate	12	12	12	12	26
Sugars, natural & added (g)	11	11	11	11	25
Fiber (g)	0	0	0	0	1
Total Fat (g)	0	2	5	8	3
Calories from Fat	11	21	43	72	22
Saturated Fat (g)	1	2	3	5	2
Trans Fat (g)	0.0	0.1	0.2	0.3	n/a
Cholesterol	8	12	22	35	8
Cholesterol (% DV)	3	4	7	12	3
Sodium	118	118	118	118	152
Potassium (mg)	383	383	383	383	425
Potassium (% DV)	11	11	11	11	12
Vitamin A (IU)	48	92	184	313	490
Vitamin A (% DV)	1	2	4	6	10
Vitamin C (mg)		2	2	2	2
Vitamin C (% DV)		4	4	4	3
Vitamin D	—	—	—	—	—
Calcium (mg)	285	285	285	285	288
Calcium (% DV)	29	29	29	29	29
Iron (mg)	0.1	0.1	0.1	0.1	0.1

	Fat-free	Low-fat 1%	Reduced-fat 2%	Whole	Chocolate 1%
Iron (% DV)	1	1	1	1	3
Phosphorus (mg)	223	223	223	223	258
Phosphorus (% DV)	22	22	22	22	26
Magnesium (mg)	27	27	27	24	32
Magnesium (% DV)	7	7	7	6	8
Vitamin B_{12}12 (mcg)	1.3	1.07	1.12	1.07	0.85
Vitamin B_{12} (% DV)	54	45	47	45	35

*Vitamin D–fortified milk can be an excellent source of vitamin D; however, levels in milk vary considerably. Read the food label or contact manufacturer for specific levels.

*Values are calculated from percent fat and percent solids— not fat of milk—using minimal California and national standards for fat-free 1 percent, 2 percent, and whole milk. Actual values may vary.

(*Courtesy:* Dairy Council of California.)

A WHOLE LATTE LOVE

Coffee Lattes—coffee made with milk—can be confusing in Latte-land if you're ordering it or making it yourself. Skinny Lattes are for the weight conscious (skim milk has less fat and calories), and Soy Lattes are it if you don't eat anything linked with eyes, since soy comes from soy beans. (Soy milk has about the same amount of protein as cow's milk and is low in saturated fat and cholesterol.) It takes a little know-how to make the perfect latte. Here are five quickie rules on how to do it, straight from Matthew Putman of Coffee.org, who prefers soy but also likes half-and-half.

- If it's just a latte you can steam any milk and it should work.
- When preparing milk for a latte, it is steamed rather than frothed,

so you're just heating up the milk, and also creating a cap of foam from the natural aeration during the steaming.

- The best milk depends on what you like. Lattes are very simple, you just need the right equipment (espresso machine with foam wand) to make a really good one.
- However, if you're making a cappuccino you'll need the traditional 50 to 50 foam milk blend, so it helps to have a dairy product that foams up good.
- Most people agree that the thicker the milk the better, so heavy cream (half-and-half) is what most coffeehouses use.

How Do You Take It?

Not all coffee lovers love lattes or cappuccinos. Some sip their java black or with milk—the healthiest way for health-conscious people. But we live in a coffee world where there is sugar, creamers, artificial sweeteners, syrups, and whipped cream—and taste buds differ from one country to another.

In Austria, whipped cream is a Coffee-mate followed by a glass of water. Middle Easterners turn to cardamom and other spices to add to their java. Salt is an Ethiopian preference. Milk in the A.M. hours and black with sugar after lunch and dinner is the way Cubans take their coffee.[2]

Coffee trivia also tells us that 30 percent of coffee drinkers in America sweeten up their cup of jolt with sugar or another sweetener. In the UK, more than 57 percent of coffee consumers turn to a sweetener, too. In India, it is commonplace to find coffee with both milk and sugar added.[3]

The Coffee Buzz on Sweet Treats

Candy: If coffee isn't available, hard coffee candies are not too difficult to find, but to find a good one is a challenge. One brand, Matlow's Hard Coffee Candy, found on the Internet at Oh! Nuts is coffee sweet and it's one that you'd be pleased to offer friends, family, and yourself.

Coffee Cakes: These sweet old-fashioned cakes are paired with drinking coffee, traced to centuries ago, a time when coffee cakes were made from scratch. Gourmet coffee cakes, like Miss Ellie's from Coffee.org (ordered online), are ones for everyday coffee cake lovers to sharing at an event—a special occasion. The last one I feasted on was the Cinnamon Walnut. As the company's description notes, "Walnut cake is unbelievably moist and absolutely addictive." This is true. It must be the farm-fresh eggs, pure bourbon vanilla, and rich sour cream that made it an extraordinary coffee cake. Yes, it is better than home-made.

Coffee Ice Cream: Drinking coffee with coffee cake is not uncommon, nor is coffee in calcium-rich ice creams. However, not all coffee ice creams win my approval. Some use artificial ingredients. Others are all natural. As a die-hard fan of Häagen-Dazs and coffee addict, I was pleased to discover there is more than one type of coffee ice cream to enjoy, especially since it was ice cream that led me into the world of coffee.

The Coffee Five ice cream contains a mere five simple ingredients: Cream, Skim Milk, Sugar, Egg Yolks, Coffee. Also, Brazilian coffee beans are given credit for the rich flavor. And yes, this coffee does contain 29 milligrams of caffeine per 1/2 cup serving, 270 calories. Not to forget some vitamin A and calcium. Häagen-Dazs offers other ice-cream flavors, including Coffee, Java Chip, and frozen coffee yogurt (I couldn't find this one in my town)—it promises less calories and more calcium and more of a jolt with its caffeine.

Coffee Yogurt: Coffee is used as a sweetener in some yogurts. They contain less sugar and less artificial ingredients than yogurts with fruit. Also, plain Greek yogurt with a bit of your favorite coffee is a wholesome treat, especially if you add fresh fruit and a cup of brew.

COFFEE AND CHOCOLATE

Coffee and chocolate are both superfoods that have been used and enjoyed for centuries. Pairing the two foods (each given a bad rap and now on the "good" for you food list) in beverages and foods can give you a double dose of antioxidants. And coffee drinking like Belgians do, with chocolate, is for chocolate lovers.

This sweet team has been paired for centuries. These days, we know both foods—separate and together—can help enhance the immune system, lower the risk of heart disease, cancer, diabetes, even obesity, and boost longevity. What's more, both supersweets can relieve dozens of ailments as well as boost energy for both work and play—and these activities can also trigger feel-good endorphins in your body.

Coffee and chocolate have a lot in common, especially if it's quality dark chocolate and quality coffee. Both once "forbidden" foods—because they contain "bad" components, including caffeine—play a role in a heart-healthy-type Mediterranean diet and lifestyle.

While I enjoyed coffee candy, ice cream, and yogurt, it's the coffee chocolates, from bars to truffles, that are unforgettable. Chocolate companies, especially the gourmet superstars that I contacted, know the power of coffee and chocolate, and look at some of the treats they've created.

Enjou Chocolat: Enjou's truffles are bite-sized chocolate confections, made with a chocolate ganache center. Their truffle collections include mocha and cappuccino. Milk chocolate truffles are 68 percent cocoa and dark chocolate truffles are 72 percent cocoa. And it doesn't stop there. Ever try Chocolate Covered Espresso Beans? These sophisticated dark chocolate coffee beans will wow coffee lovers.

Fran's Chocolates: Like Enjou Chocolat, Fran's offers truffles, too. As the description of their dark chocolate espresso truffles notes, "locally roasted Café vita espresso is infused into fresh organic cream, and then carefully stirred into dark couverture (a French term meaning a glossy, coated chocolate)." This combination brings on an unforgettable and intense dark chocolate espresso experience, thanks to the espresso-infused cream being dipped into 64 percent dark couverture.

The ingredients in these espresso truffles are ones I can pronounce, like dark chocolate, cocoa beans, sugar, cocoa butter, soy lecithin, vanilla, organic cream, invert sugar, organic butter, and coffee beans. It's the same story for the milk chocolate espresso truffles, but that cream is dipped into 38 percent milk couverture after dark for a strong café au lait experience. Both truffles are rich, creamy gems that paired with a cup of coffee are bliss.

Fran's Story: Chocolates 'n' Coffee

Meet Fran, a woman behind fine chocolate. Back in 1982, Fran introduced the artisan chocolate experience for consumers when she opened her European-style chocolate shop in Seattle, Washington.

Created as a place to showcase her sublimely rich desserts, Fran's shop also offered caramels and truffles, which quickly captured the favor of her customers and became her signature confections. Her best-selling gray salt and smoked salt caramels, and caramels covered in dark and milk chocolate, are classic favorites. . . . And I have had the pleasure to savor both and sip coffee—all types—with the chocolate caramels.

Many of Fran's products have been recognized by the National Association of Specialty Food: the gray and smoked salt caramels were each awarded a Gold Medal for Outstanding Confection and the dark hot chocolate was awarded the Gold Medal for Outstanding Hot Beverage. What's more, these days, Fran's uses the same Café vita espresso at their stores for all their coffee drinks: espressos, Americanos, lattes, mochas, and more.

Fran, chocolatier extraordinaire, knows the true power of the chocolate and coffee connection. She told me, "I believe chocolate and coffee are a perfect pairing, each enhances the other." Fran added, "They grow in the same areas—the coffee on the hillsides and the cocoa trees below. They share the same terroir. And this is what makes them so complementary to each other."

(*Courtesy:* Fran's Story: franschocolate.com.)

MarieBelle: When I opened the blue box of MarieBelle chocolates I sensed I was in for a decadent chocolate coffee adventure. Three chocolates wooed me as I read their descriptions in a fold-out brochure. I nibbled and read the words: "Kona Bean: The white chocolate ganache (a blend of the finest Belgian chocolate, cream, sweet butter, and natural flavorings) is mixed with actual grains of Hawaiian Kona coffee and covered with chocolate. Coffee: The milk chocolate ganache is made with fresh roasted, ground arabica coffee beans. Espresso: A dark chocolate ganache infused with 100 percent Arabica beans resulting in a strikingly dark tasting chocolate with a profound coffee flavor." And that's not all. . . .

Vosges: Enter an exotic chocolate bar. Creole Exotic Candy Bar: "This dark chocolate, rich in flavonoids, holds the zip of chicory coffee that lifts you before you even sink your teeth in and feel the crunch of cocoa nibs." I'm talking about a New Orleans style chicory coffee and bittersweet chocolate (70 percent cacao). This isn't a mass-market quick-fix candy bar. It's a decadent bar that you'll savor and taste the layers of coffee and chocolate.

Homemade chocolate coffee desserts are a treasure year-round. This rich soy chocolate coffee mousse recipe is made at a California spa and dished up to spa goers.

Dark Chocolate Mousse

❖ ❖ ❖

16 ounces silken tofu
4 ounces bittersweet
    chocolate, chopped
⅓ cup cocoa powder

½ cup decaffeinated coffee
1 cup agave
1 teaspoon vanilla extract

In a food processor or blender, puree the tofu until smooth. Place the chopped chocolate, cocoa powder, and coffee in a saucepan. Stir constantly over medium-low heat until melted and smooth. Remove from heat and mix in the agave and vanilla. Stir until smooth. Add chocolate mixture to tofu and puree until well blended. Put in bowl and chill at least two hours. To serve, scoop one quarter-cup of mousse onto plate and surround with berries. Serves 12.

(*Courtesy:* Christine Denny, Food Services Director; The Oaks at Ojai.)

Speaking of sweet coffee combos, in part 5, "The Ultimate Brew," you'll learn that incorporating coffee into your diet and lifestyle can help you get and/or stay lean as well as add years to your life. The healing powers of coffee are becoming known by coffee lovers as part of a superfood that is essential to maintaining your weight, staying healthy, stalling age-related diseases, and living a longer, quality life—and you'll find out exactly how it can do that.

A Cup Full of Perks

✓ Adding milk in your cup of java adds calcium, protein, and other good-for-you nutrients.

✓ Beware of coffee products, including candy and ice cream, which flaunt "includes coffee," because it can often be an artificial flavoring and not real java. And see where coffee ranks on the product label. The closer to being the first ingredient, the more coffee.

✓ Both coffee and dark chocolate have been found to contain anti-oxidants—compounds that are linked to heart health, lowering risk of developing cancers, and boosting longevity.

✓ Pairing the right chocolate with the right coffee in desserts is an experience that is exciting for your taste buds and overall health and well-being.

PART 5

THE ULTIMATE BREW

CHAPTER 10

The Skinny Beverage

Coffee is a beverage that puts one to sleep when not drank.
—Alphonse Allais, French writer, humorist
(1854–1905)[1]

My college and coffee days came with semester breaks. During one period, I was living a Bohemian lifestyle in Hollywood, Southern California. I worked at 24-hour coffee shops as a waitress. The work kept me and my dog fed and the rent paid—and kept unwanted pounds off. One weekend I escaped L.A. with my roommate and canine companion for a beautifying desert minivacation.

We left Los Angeles for Palm Springs—a desert haven—to get sun, fun, and dump five pounds with ease. In the morning, I woke up to a 12-ounce cup of regular brew (no Double-Double with double sugar and double cream and No Whip). It gave me energy to pool hop, going from one hotel pool to another. It even gave me the brainstorm to sneak my water-loving dog, a black Lab, Stone Fox, into the cold water, too. During the afternoon I tasted my first cold coffee drink. I ordered it at a café for the rich. One iced café mocha—and cold water to go for my pooch. Not only did the chocolaty coffee flavor and temperature of the sweet beverage cool me down, but the caffeine gave me more physical energy and zapped hunger pangs so I could continue to play and swim, enjoying the long days of leisure.

These days, at Lake Tahoe, I get my morning wake-up jolt from hot coffee—all kinds. It gives me motivation to stay active and keep balanced. Teamed with the Mediterranean diet and lifestyle, coffee works to keep moving. It's the Mediterranean foods, the pools where I swim—and coffee in moderation—that keep me from looking like a middle-aged spayed feline. I feel more like a healthy coffee plant, but nourishing myself. But eating right and drinking coffee to keep off unwanted pounds is nothing new.

EAT LESS, DRINK MORE JAVA JUICE . . .

Since biblical times, the health conscious have turned to juice fasting for its body-cleansing and weight-loss benefits. Natural fruits and vegetables flush toxins from your body. And they flush away fat, too. What's more, coffee can speed up the weight loss.

Eating this way isn't just about weight loss; it's about cleaning out your digestive system. You'll not only feel thinner; you'll also feel positively thinner.

Enter the Grapefruit Diet. From the thirties on into the fifties, Hollywood dieters have turned to the slimming power of this wonder citrus—and coffee.

The grapefruit's status as the ideal diet food was born when researchers found evidence that it contains fat-dissolving compounds. Further elevating the fruit's status in the world of weight loss: It's low cal, fat-free, fiber rich, vitamin packed, and satisfying.

What You Eat: On this regimen, the day's menu includes $1/2$ grapefruit and black coffee for breakfast; $1/2$ grapefruit, 1 hard-boiled egg, 1 cucumber, 1 dry melba toast, and coffee for lunch; and 1 whole grapefruit, 2 hard-boiled eggs, $1/2$ head lettuce, 1 tomato, and coffee for dinner.

Why You'll Love It: Grapefruit and hard-boiled eggs are the quintessential diet foods. Eating them lets your brain know that you've pulled out the stops.

- Grapefruit: One medium grapefruit has just 74 calories, less than 1 gram of fat, and it is a good source of fiber.
- Eggs: One medium-boiled egg has only 69 calories. Try eating just the hard-cooked egg white—it's low in fat and calories and high in the amino acid cysteine, a skin-supporting nutrient.
- Coffee: Plus, the coffee—black—acts as an appetite suppressant, making this plan easier to stick with.
  Tips: Consult your doctors before starting this or any weight-loss regimen. Drink six to eight 8-ounce glasses of water daily (including coffee). Use spices such as cinnamon to enhance the flavor of grapefruit and vinegar for vegetables.

THE 21ST-CENTURY SECRET TO COFFEE AND CELLULITE

Minifasts like the Grapefruit Diet and exercise can help to detox your body and lessen the appearance of cellulite, aka unwanted dimpled body fat. Dermatologists will tell you that more than 90 percent of women are plagued by cellulite—not surprising, since formation of the characteristic dimpled-looking flesh is tied to estrogen, as well as genetics, age, processed food, lack of water, and a sedentary lifestyle.

But that doesn't mean you can't do something about it. Health experts recommend the following strategies to shrink cellulite.

Getting rid of water weight: Water-dense foods—including coffee—act as natural diuretics to help eliminate excess water, which can make dimpled fat look less pronounced.

Eating high-fiber foods: Fiber-rich foods—yes, coffee contains dietary fiber—can help eliminate waste and toxins from your body and prevent a buildup of fat and water.

Burning off calories: To burn fat and tone up, coffee provides the motivation to get a move on.

Water loss: Caffeine in coffee can act as a natural diuretic, increasing the amount of urine you'll excrete by temporarily losing pounds or water weight—but it does not get rid of body fat. And that's where anti-cellulite, fat-burning foods come into play.

The Anticellulite Book That Changed My Life

In my twenties, I remember reading a book about beating cellulite. The rules included that one must stay clear from chocolate and coffee. That didn't work for me or my lifestyle. Just the thought of a life without these two "bad" foods was enough for me to toss the book.

But I kept physically active, ate lots of fresh fruits and vegetables, and drank water. I didn't dump coffee, either. After all, a feel-good caffeine fix is what helped to motivate me to exercise, making my time at the gym and outdoors walking and swimming last longer—and I enjoyed it.

Over time, I learned that it's a challenge to get rid of lumpy body fat, whether you're lean or overweight. Cellulite also appears more as you age, but you can reduce the appearance of the stuff. So, I follow a healthful diet and lifestyle (no smoking or overindulging in alcohol), keep fit, and pass on "Thunder Thighs"—a double-tall mocha made with whole milk with extra whipped cream (except on superspecial occasions).

HOW COFFEE DRINKERS STAY SLIM

Spa nutritionists will tell you that drinking a soothing hot beverage, including tea and coffee, is similar to having a hot cup of soup before a meal. It satisfies your appetite and you'll eat less. A hot liquid can fill you up, not out.

Coffee—regular and decaf—is served at health spas around the globe. Some of the best coffees help women and men get and stay slim because they contain caffeine, antioxidants, and dietary fiber, and coffee is a natural diuretic that can help stimulate water loss—and/or beat bloat as well as keep you regular. Then, if you turn to the weight loss coffee superstar—a known fat fighter in moderation—you'll be on the path to real weight loss.

But note, it's a cup of regular coffee that can help you lose the unwanted pounds and body fat—not the added fun junk added to coffee beverages. That means, stay clear of specialty coffee drinks with added cream, flavored syrups, whipped cream, half-and-half, and whole milk. It's tempting to order a Grande (16-ounce coffee complete with all the frills). But if you want to maintain your ideal weight, go coffee au naturel.

If you're trying to keep your weight in check, tasty coffee creamers are another lure for coffee lovers. Coffee creamers (nondairy and reduced fat) can spell extra fat and calories. And the nutritional labels on these flavoring can be mind boggling. One teaspoon may be a mere 10 calories and zero fat. But in reality, how many people follow directions (especially if it's a yummy-flavored Coffee-mate)? So, the end result can be dozens of calories and saturated fat—the kind that clogs your arteries and sabotages a healthful cup of black coffee.

So, if you want to stay on the skinny track, keep it real: regular coffee with a splash of low-fat or skim milk and natural flavorings, such as a dash of cinnamon or cocoa powder.

Not only can drinking the right coffee help you to lose water weight, but the soothing beverage can both calm and uplift your spirits. Coffee breaks give you a minivacation to replenish your body, mind, and spirit. Take a look at the easy-to-whip-up DIY recipe on page 128 that'll help you to chill and keep those pounds at bay during spring, summer, or on vacation. Speaking of vacations, from minifasts to detox diets and methods can help you to cleanse your body, which can help give you a jump-start on feeling energized and losing unwanted pounds and body fats.

THE LEGENDARY COFFEE ENEMA

Welcome to the coffee enema, a detoxing method that has been used in the past and present. Years ago, when I was writing diet articles for *Woman's World* magazine, I recall interviewing someone at a popular Southern California health spa. I was invited to visit and have a complimentary coffee enema. A bit skittish, I passed (no pun intended). These days, while it does seem intriguing, I prefer to detox my system with water, herbal teas, and plenty of organic fruits and vegetables. But other people, maybe even you, may consider the coffee enema. Please consult with your health practitioner before you try a coffee enema, as it is a controversial procedure, but one that is touted by many health practitioners.

Enter Ann Louise Gittleman, Ph.D.: "The most overlooked value of coffee is its use in the legendary coffee enema. It turns out that coffee has been proven to increase an enzyme known as Glutahione S-transferase or GST—which elevates the uptake of gluthathione by 700 percent. That means GST activates glutathione to bind to toxins—making them water-soluble for excretion," she explains.

Gittleman adds, "Coffee helps to dilate blood vessels and bile ducts to remove toxic overload more efficiently." This, in turn, can help us get rid of a "plethora of environmental assaults," including pesticides, prescription meds, and preservatives.

Before you start, Gittleman advises using organic coffee, made fresh the night before, and cooled down. While any enema or douche bag can be used, she recommends the Kendall Seamless Enema Bucket (available at a medical supply house or the Kendall Company). Then, you're good to go, so to speak. Here is a 10-step recipe, straight from the good doctor Gittleman.

Coffee Enema Recipe

1. Pour one quart of pure water into a glass, stainless steel, or enamel coffee maker (never aluminum or Teflon-coated). Add three tablespoons ground coffee. The amount of coffee that you used depends on your tolerance for caffeine. Start with a weak coffee enema rather than a strong one. Percolated coffee is also acceptable.

2. Hang the enema bag no higher than two feet off the floor. Hanging it any higher causes the fluid to flow out with too much force.

3. Connect the colon tube to the enema bag and seal off the tube.

4. Pour the coffee into the enema bag and allow a little to pour from the end of the tube into the toilet or container in order to clear air from the tube. This is also a good time to recheck the temperature of the coffee to make sure it's not too hot.

5. Lubricate several inches of the free end of the colon tube and insert it into the rectum, while lying on your left side. The length of tubing inserted varies greatly with individuals. Never try to force the tubing in. Expect to take several enemas before you become comfortable with the procedure.

6. Unseal the tube and control the flow of coffee into the colon.

7. When the flow is completed, remove the colon tube or leave it in place with the valve open to remove gas that may be in the colon.

8. Gently massage your abdomen for five minutes, while lying on your left side. Do the same while lying on your back, and then on your right side.

9. After 15 minutes, sit on the toilet and expel the enema. Should you wish to do so at any time before this, do not hesitate. You should never try to forcibly hold in the enema. In fact, nothing in this entire procedure should involve force or strain.

10. I would recommend that you start with one coffee enema per week and see how you do. If you feel headachy, depressed, or even constipated, these are signs your body is trying to move out toxins and you should proceed slowly, but surely. Simply put, the coffee enema is starting to clear layers of waste from your system. They are best administered in the morning as sometimes the caffeine can keep you awake at night. Take the enema after a bowel movement rather than before one.[2]

POUNDS-OFF, COFFEE-FLAVORED ICE

Susan Terkel shares her original and sweet coffee secret that helped her shed unwanted weight:

My favorite coffee recipe is for Spanish Granita, to be served between courses (to cleanse the palate): 3 cups espresso coffee plus a few tablespoons (I use 2 or 3) of liquor—coffee brandy or just brandy—zest of lemon and zest of orange; 1/3 cup of sugar. Freeze, then shave with a fork and serve in a glass dish, such as a champagne flute—after the main course and before dessert.

A variation of this, which I make more than that, is to add 2 cups of milk to the coffee (and I admit that I used a sugar substitute). I eat that whenever I have the munchies and lost about 15 to 20 pounds one year—just relying on my Coffee Granita.

Once you get into the groove of drinking coffee to help you maintain your ideal weight, like me, Susan, and countless other women and men do, it will be easy and rewarding. Still, you have to be coffee savvy or you'll unwittingly be adding hidden calories and fat. Forego sugar, cream, and syrups that are used in those pretty coffees. (But go ahead and splurge on occasion.) Lose the idea of teaming high-fat, high-calorie doughnuts or hamburgers when you order a coffee "with legs."

Learn to enjoy coffee for coffee. If you can make the switcheroo and drop the coffee extras you'll also drop 300 to 600 calories.

Iced Coffee with Honey

❖ ❖ ❖

Use 1 cup coffee. Pour over cracked ice, or ice cubes, with 1 teaspoon honey, into a glass. Dust with ground cinnamon and ground nutmeg. Serves 1.

(*Courtesy:* The Roast and Post Coffee Company; www.realcoffee.co.uk.)

So drinking Go-Juice in moderation to help you to stay physical and maintain your ideal weight can work, which can help you to stay healthier and age more gracefully. In chapter 11, "Antiaging Toast to Life," you'll get another buzz on the power of coffee. Mother Nature's superfood coffee in many ways can stall Father Time and add years to your life.

A CUP FULL OF PERKS

✓ Coffee and grapefruit contain fat-burning benefits to help you lose unwanted pounds and body fat.
✓ In moderation coffee can help you to lessen the appearance of cellulite.
✓ Keeping your cup(s) of java pure (without lots of artificial flavorings, sugar, and creamers) can help you get and stay slim.
✓ Coffee enemas are used at spas as a way of detoxing the body, which can be energizing and have immediate weight loss effects.
✓ Coffee and honey pairing provides a double dose of antioxidants and superfoods to provide extra energy to help you exercise (burning calories and boosting metabolism at rest) and help to stave off muscle aches and pain after a workout.

Antiaging Toast to Life

I have measured out my life with coffee spoons.
—T.S. Eliot[1]

During my life, coffee continued to be part of my days and nights, and my friend during life's ups and downs. When I was 25, my mother passed at 52. I was heartbroken, as was her mother, my grandmother Adele (of Osage Indian roots). I promised I would bring my mother's box of ashes to her. And coffee was part of the trek to help me stay awake and stay strong.

So like the classic song "A Horse with No Name" I set out on a Greyhound bus through the desert wasteland to Tucson, Arizona. On this road trip coffee—regular roast—at coffee shops throughout my rides helped me accomplish my mission. It was coffee that helped uplift my spirit and keep me alert as we traveled more than 1,500 miles round-trip on a family mission.

I arrived at Gran's condo in a high-rise building. The woman, at 75 both mentally and physically healthy, had a fresh pot of Colombian coffee sitting on the kitchen counter. A package of butter cookies was next to the brew. Against a mountain backdrop with cactus plants outside, we talked in the living room.

Flashbacks about my mom, once a strong, hardworking, intelligent woman with Osage Indian roots, were the topic of our conversation while we sipped coffee. The hot beverage was comforting and gave me extra mental and physical energy to talk and nurture my gran. This was one of many dangling coffee chats we shared—with the sweetness of "Mother's little helper" and cookies.

COFFEE AND BRAIN WELLNESS

Researchers have shown coffee lovers that both regular and decaf roasts may be linked to the brain. In fact, coffee may help to stave off brain conditions such as Alzheimer's, Parkinson's, dementia, and depression—problems that affect people more as they age.

Alzheimer's disease: Researchers have gone to the drawing board more than once to figure out if there is a connection between coffee and lowering the risk of Alzheimer's disease (a brain disease that affects proper brain function and whose symptoms include memory loss and confusion).

Past and present research shows coffee is not to be ignored when it comes to matters of the mind. One study published in the *European Journal of Neurology* analyzed the link between caffeine in coffee and protection against the degeneration of the brain that is connected with Alzheimer's disease (AD) in the early stages. The end result: More research is needed to detect if caffeine is the component that may protect people by helping to keep nerves in the brain from breaking down.[2]

But it's not just caffeine that may lower the risk of developing Alzheimer's. Another compound may work with caffeine and protect against this disease that affects the brain. One finding, for instance, shows that caffeinated coffee induces an increase in blood levels of a growth factor GCSF (granulocyte colony stimulating factor). Researchers note that moderate coffee drinking (4 to 5 cups per day) starting in middle age—and it's never too late—may provide protection for Alzheimer's symptoms and disease.[3]

How It Works: Caffeine and other "mystery" compounds may be the clue to how coffee can stave off Alzheimer's disease. More research is needed before it's the prescription of choice. Still, drinking coffee cannot hurt and it may be worth the time and effort for people to turn to the healthful beverage.

Parkinson's disease: Like with the scourge of Alzheimer's, coffee drinkers may also be less likely to develop Parkinson's (a brain disease that destroys the brain cells that affect an individual's ability to move). Symptoms include slowness of movement and trembling. In the United States, at least 500,000 people suffer from Parkinson's; the average onset is about 60 (slightly more common in men) and increases with age, according to sobering numbers from the National Institute of Neurological Disorders and Stroke.

A past study published in the *Journal of the American Medical Association*, an ambitious work using coffee and monitoring more than 8,000 Japanese-American men who put it to work, found that higher coffee and caffeine intake is linked with lower odds of developing Parkinson's disease. The results hint that it's the caffeine and not other nutrients in coffee that deserve credit.[4]

How It Works: It may be the caffeine in coffee that deserves credit for the good news about less chance of developing Parkinson's, but chocolate and soft drinks (which also contain caffeine) have not panned out with the same positive results. More research is needed, but caffeine may hold one of the keys to staving off this disease that affects millions of people.

What You Can Do: Drinking coffee can help you to de-stress, especially if you enjoy a cup of java in a social setting or solo in a relaxing environment. Coffee after a lunch or dinner including the "brain food" fish (high in essential fatty acids) is what brain wellness doctors order, for preventive measures. Eating more antioxidant-rich vegetables—and antioxidant-rich coffee—will help get rid of free radicals, which may help brain health, too.

COFFEE AND STROKE

People of all ages have strokes. But the older you are, the greater your risk for stroke. The odds of having a stroke, notes the American Heart Association, more than doubles for each decade of life after age 55. But coffee drinkers, like me, who aren't getting any younger, may be pleasantly surprised that their daily cup of joe could be of help.

Researchers at Harvard and from the Universidad Autónoma de Madrid looked at the link between coffee and strokes in women. Coffee does stimulate the heart, so medical doctors and nutritionists, past and present, say that too much coffee might be a bad thing for heart health. But get this—a study showed that's not exactly true. The Nurses' Health Study, tracked 83,000 women who completed food-related questionnaires, including questions about their personal coffee drinking, for 24 years. Scientists discovered that women who drank two or three cups of coffee a day reduced their risk of stroke by 19 percent. Women who did not smoke cigarettes reported even greater benefits.[5]

How It Works: This study backs up the hypothesis that components—not caffeine—may be the good guys and provide a guard effect for stroke. Add the *Dr. Chopra Says* authors: "Coffee, like wine, has hundreds of component chemicals, including potassium, magnesium, vitamin E, and antioxidants."[6]

What You Can Do: No, drinking coffee is not the silver bullet, but it can help you to put an antistroke package together. Drinking antioxidant-rich coffee in moderation will help you to feel energized, so you're more likely to get a move on and exercise regularly. That means, both exercise and revving up your metabolism will help you to maintain your ideal weight, which can help you to keep your blood pressure down. Also, if you take a "coffee break" it will help you to rest and relax—two keys to help you de-stress and keep you more balanced as well as focused, so problem solving can be easier and not lead to losing your cool.

COFFEE AND STALLING FATHER TIME

Disease and health challenges, whether they be Parkinson's or stroke, increase as we age, but that doesn't mean we are helpless.

Research continues to turn up more and more health benefits for coffee—a real bonus for coffee drinkers.[7]

Risk of Parkinson's: Drops 40 percent

Risk of Type 2 Diabetes: Drops 28–54 percent

Risk of Colorectal Cancer: Drops 24–48 percent

Risk of Liver Cirrhosis: Drops 22–40 percent

Studies have found at least 10 different health benefits for coffee, including:

1. Coffee increases alertness and mental performance.
2. Coffee helps relieve bronchial asthma symptoms.

3. Coffee improves short-term memory.
4. Coffee increases endurance and sports performance.
5. Coffee reduces Parkinson's disease.
6. Coffee reduces the risk of type 2 diabetes.
7. Coffee reduces the risk of Alzheimer's disease.
8. Coffee prevents the formation of gallstones.
9. Coffee reduces the risk of cirrhosis of the liver.
10. Coffee reduces the risk of colorectal cancer and liver cancer.

Long Live One Grounded Baker-ess

Several years ago, I was introduced to Gemma, an upbeat, down-to-earth woman who was behind the man of the grassroots of olive oil production. Her late husband, Joseph, began Nick Sciabica & Sons, a family-run business. Both Joseph and Gemma, residents of Modesto, California, followed the traditional Mediterranean diet and lifestyle.

Last year, Joseph, 95, passed on—just five years away from becoming a 100-year-old-man. (The average lifespan of men in America is 74.) As I wrote in *The Healing Powers of Olive Oil*, "Joseph isn't overweight, doesn't have high blood pressure or cholesterol, nor does Gemma." Indeed, this couple were my role models and for good reason. I believe he lived 20 years longer than his peers for a variety of reasons: a happy marriage, loving family, a sense of self, and accomplishments—and maybe his intake of coffee, too.

I remember Gemma telling me in one of our countless telephone conversations that both she and Joseph every morning drank a cup of coffee sweetened with honey. So, while he didn't make it to 100, it was close. So if one follows the Mediterranean diet and lifestyle—including coffee in moderation—good health and a quality life, like Joseph enjoyed, may be the end result.

METABOLIC SYNDROME

If you're middle-aged, like me, you may be spooked by this all-too-common syndrome, which is a deadly combo of risk factors, including high blood pressure, high blood sugar, unhealthy cholesterol levels, and too much belly fat. And the scourge of metabolic syndrome hits home for millions of people in America and around the globe.

These factors (often silent killers and increasing as you grow older) double your risk of developing heart disease—strokes and heart attacks—and type 2 diabetes. As I've noted in previous chapters, those facing these health risks can benefit from coffee as a preventive measure. Coffee indeed can help lower your risk of becoming another heart disease statistic.

Past research touts coffee's polyphenols—again. Researchers have discovered that water extracts of roasted coffee residues, including coffee antioxidants caffeic acid and chlorogenic acid, are the superstars responsible for coffee's good metabolic effects. But it doesn't stop there.

Sure, drinking coffee in moderation can help lower your risk of becoming another walking wounded of metabolic syndrome, but so can lifestyle changes. Go back to chapter 6 and get familiar with the Mediterranean diet and lifestyle. Medical researchers show that fewer vegetarians than meat eaters have metabolic syndrome, thanks to a plant-based diet. Get a move on every day, too, so you can maintain a healthy weight, fitness, and well-being. This, in turn, can help you get and/or stay healthy and live a longer, quality life, as Joseph Sciabica did.

The Power Lift

❖ ❖ ❖

1½ cups brewed coffee, cold or at room temperature
2 medium ripe bananas, peeled and sliced
2 tablespoons honey, or to taste

2 6-ounce containers plain low-fat yogurt (1½ cups)
3 to 4 ice cubes
2 tablespoons toasted wheat germ

Use more or less honey depending on the ripeness of the bananas. Place all ingredients in a blender container. Cover, and blend on high speed for 1 minute, or until smooth. Pour into 4 glasses. Serve immediately. Makes four 8-ounce servings.

(*Courtesy:* Coffee Science Source.)

Scientists and doctors are leaning toward a verdict that says "yes," coffee increases better health and longevity. Both regular and decaf get credit. While java may boost lifespan, it makes sense to enjoy the other benefits of coffee that can help lessen a wide variety of pesky health ailments, which you can put to use right now, as you'll discover in the next chapter, brimming over with home cures.

A Cup Full of Perks

✓ Coffee can help feed your brain to lower the risk of developing age-related Alzheimer's and Parkinson's, thanks to its caffeine.

✓ It may be the multiple compounds in coffee that can help lower the odds of developing a stroke.

✓ Metabolic syndrome is the scourge for boomers and the elderly, but drinking coffee in moderation can help keep blood pressure, cholesterol, blood sugar, and belly fat in check and under control.

✓ Coffee can boost longevity in conjunction with a healthful diet and lifestyle.

PART 6

COFFEE CURES

1 2

Home Remedies from Your Kitchen

As soon as coffee is in your stomach, there is a general commotion. Ideas begin to move . . . similes arise, the paper is covered. Coffee is your ally and writing ceases to be a struggle.
—Honoré de Balzac (1799–1859)[1]

After my journey through the desert I ended up back on campus—a place like a field of beans where growing and processing of coffee starts. The big challenge in my senior year was to write 100 pages of creative writing to be judged whether I was creative enough to be accepted as a graduate student in the creative writing department at San Francisco State. I turned to brain juice to create creative non-fiction—stories and poetry.

On a hot spring day, I woke up in the San Jose suburbs (again), but this time I—not my mother—made the coffee. Living in a large blue house with landscaped yards (much like the one I grew up in as a kid), I shared it with two Labrador retrievers and one cat. With piles of papers throughout each room in the house I wrote and rewrote my words—and coffee was my constant companion (again).

Sipping the instant generic stuff in the morning and visiting coffee shops in the afternoon, I put together, bit by bit, poems and prose. It's the coffee power—or caffeine kick—that enhanced my brainpower and got me through the writing process and into the graduate program. In retrospect, I was like a coffee bean passing the quality check during the handpicking to grading process during harvest time. And that's not all. . . .

During this chapter of my life, I turned to coffee for its variety of perks. I drank coffee to help me get through bouts of irregularity (thanks to being a sedentary student with an erratic diet and schedule). The coffee helped stave off PMS crankies and cramps—both woes I was challenged with as I traveled 100 miles three times a week to go to college and get a degree so I could sit here and write for a living (and drink more java to meet deadlines).

Discovering home cures, like these, can help you get to where you want to go—and often home cures work to cure common ailments, which will make you a believer that coffee does have healing powers.

Also, since coffee contains caffeine, it can give you a feel-good, energizing buzz, and because the magical beans can help cure what's ailing you, it can give you a sense of well-being or natural "high" or "buzz" (a word in slang dictionaries) like seeing the Colorado Rocky Mountains, the Washington coast, or the aqua blue ocean of the Florida Keys.

Read on, and you'll see why coffee is a versatile brew that you want to have in your pantry and savor in each and every room, to heal yourself. Turn to chapter 7 to discover different types of coffee roasts and how to make espresso drinks and chapter 8 for flavored coffees.

CURES FROM YOUR KITCHEN

I'll describe 50 common health ailments from A to Z and provide why there is a growing trend about at-home coffee cures that'll get you buzzed. I include tried-and-tested folk remedies (some sound, some quirky), scientific studies, and medical experts' words of coffee smarts—and my own experiences with ailments treated with coffee. Meet the different roasts, blends, flavored coffees, and drinks that can be your best friend. But caution: Consult your health-care practitioner before putting to work any coffee cure.

1 **AGOROPHOBIA (Face the daily grind):** Ever met someone who has a fear of open spaces and prefers to stay homebound like memorable characters in films, including the traumatized shrink in *Copycat* or the reclusive author in *Finding Forrester?* Some people, like me, who work in a calm home environment, have a mild form of this phobia. (After working in a controlled space it feels like cultural shock to go to an intense grocery store when it's prime time, so I avoid doing it.) But coffee (regular with caffeine) seems to help give me a sense of wanting to get outdoors and go swimming or walk the dogs, counteracting the feelings of wanting to stay home in my comfort zone. It's like a gentle nudge to get me to go where I need to go.

What Coffee Rx to Use: Opt for an 8-ounce cup of medium-roast coffee (which does contain caffeine) or a blend of half milk and half decaf, which is similar to drinking a cup of green tea caffeine-wise. Milk, with its compound tryptophan, calms nerves.

Why You'll Be Perked Up! Not only will you get antistress antioxidants in coffee, but the caffeine fix may be just enough to give you the combo effect of motivation to go outdoors and do what you want to do, whether it be run errands, socialize, work, or exercise, and the feel-good effect. Start slowly, and if coffee works for you, the more you face the fear the more you'll desensitize yourself to facing your fear factor and survive.

2 **ASTHMA (Jump-start your breathing):** Not wanting to leave your safe haven is uncomfortable, but so is feeling like a fish out of water. The breathing difficulty of an asthma attack is the result of airway inflammation and constriction. It may be linked to allergies, stress, or a compromised immune system. Coughing, wheezing, and chest tightness can be common symptoms that'll leave you wanting a remedy—conventional or a home cure.

What Coffee Rx to Use: Drink an 8- or 12-ounce cup of antioxidant-rich medium- or dark-roast coffee in the morning as a preventative measure. Afterward, put the coffee energy to work and exercise to help healthy up your heart and lungs.

Why You'll Be Perked Up! It's believed that a cup of excellence may be just the cure for coffee lovers, since it can help open airways for those suffering from asthma. Coffee contains natural theophylline that helps stop bronchospasms and even open constricted bronchial passages. Some folk remedy wizards believe a couple cups of coffee can help you breathe better for several hours.

3 **ALLERGIES (Savor a day starter):** If asthma doesn't affect your life, allergies just might. Triggers can vary, from pollen during allergy season to substances, including dust, air pollutants, molds, and more. And symptoms, like asthma, can disrupt your life—from sinus headaches, sniffles, and coughing to nasal congestion—and can make your daily grind miserable.

What Coffee Rx to Use: Try drinking one 8-ounce cup of strong dark-roast coffee (hold the milk and cream, which can add to congestion) with 1 tablespoon of locally produced honey. Repeat as needed up to three times per day.

Why You'll Be Perked Up! By taking the coffee-honey cure, you can help the caffeine in a cup of jolt speed up the honey cure. Honey can help your body build up immunity to pollen. Some savvy beekeepers believe that your immune system will get used to the local pollen in it and won't go haywire when pollen is in the air. Not only will allergy symptoms buzz off, but due to the water you use in coffee you'll be hydrating yourself and help lessen postnasal drip. It's a double punch of Mother Nature's finest and without the side effects of over-the-counter allergy pills or prescription steroid sprays.

4 **ANXIETY (Sip a chill beverage):** While pesky allergies—all types—can haunt you, especially in the spring and fall, high anxiety can be nightmarish. Welcome to a world of tightening muscles, queasiness, headaches, and a fight-or-flight response. Anxiety can sneak up on you without warning like a great earthquake or hit like a tsunami during stressful times in life. But don't despair.

What Coffee Rx to Use: A 6-ounce or 8-ounce cup of regular coffee (half decaf or decaf) before or even during a mild wave of anxiety can calm your nerves. Go for a café au lait (French for "coffee and milk") with equal amounts of strong-brewed drip coffee and hot milk. Or try a latte—an espresso-based beverage with steamed milk. (Milk contains calming calcium and magnesium minerals.) Hold the sugar. Repeat in moderation as needed.

Why You'll Be Perked Up! Coffee—a variety of blends and types—is believed to get you wired because of its caffeine content. However, coffee has other feel-good compounds in it that can actually relax you and provide a sense of well-being.

One afternoon I was feeling stressed out and a bit tired due to life's ups and downs. Two feelings that can be the perfect setup for an anxiety attack. Instead of chamomile, I fixed a cup of coffee mocha (a latte blended with chocolate). Fifteen minutes after, I felt a sense of calm and was more grounded. I took my blood pressure and was pleasantly surprised. Both systolic and diastolic numbers were below normal—117/70/58. So next time you want to chill, try coffee (paired with milk). It's one of the least expected and fastest-working anxiety cures.

5 **ATTENTION DEFICIT DISORDER (Focus with brain juice):** Like anxiety, this disorder plagues countless people (of all ages). It's healthier to cope naturally—and it can be done. You may be thinking, "Coffee to help you focus? Give me a coffee break, right." Wrong. Actually, coffee might be the next "drug" doctors prescribe for Attention Deficit Disorder (ADD) and Attention Deficit Hyperactive Disorder (ADHD).

The Coffee Rx to Use: Take one 8-ounce cup of regular freshbrewed medium roast (it contains the most caffeine compared to other coffees). Skip sugar and flavorings.

Why You'll Be Perked Up! I believe coffee may be a good medicine in moderation because the natural brew can both help calm you and enhance concentration. Prescription drugs, such as Ritalin, aid in upping the level of the brain chemical dopamine (the same thing a caffeine buzz can do), which ends up calming an overactive mind to keep it on track.

6 **BALDNESS (Try a healthful treatment):** Losing focus can be one thing that wreaks havoc on your well-being, but watching your hair go down the drain in the shower can cause despair for both men and women. My grandfather had a receding hairline; my dad had a full head of hair; my brother is somewhere in be-

tween and chose to go for the "turtlehead" look like the popular celebs Sean Connery and Bruce Willis. But there are folk remedies to try before you grab the razor.

The Coffee Rx to Use: Drink one 8-ounce Irish coffee drink (with dark French roast and whisky). Repeat a few times per week. Once or twice daily enjoy an 8-ounce mug of medium roast.

Why You'll Be Perked Up! Scientists have proven that caffeine in coffee stimulates the growth of small follicles in the scalp of men who are suffering from hair loss. Coffee enhances the ability to resist the depleting effects of DHT (dihydrotestosterone), which is the leading cause for male baldness. A bonus: Scientists believe both medium and dark roast contain antioxidants, the good guys to help your skin and hair stay younger.[2]

7 **BLAHS (Grab a pick-me-up):** Whether hair loss is bugging you or you're simply feeling lousy for no pinpointed reason, it's a feeling you can control with a good cup (or two) of java juice. Temporary setbacks and rough patches come and go, but coffee can help give you a bounce in your walk.

What Coffee Rx to Use: One 8-ounce cappuccino in the morning and an 8-ounce au lait in the afternoon may be the perfect remedy to lift your spirits. Pair it with a dark chocolate truffle or piece of fresh fruit. Repeat as necessary. But do not overindulge, because it may create an up-and-down effect with mood swings like sugar can do.

Why You'll Be Perked Up! Make way, sugary sodas, for "One Cup of Coffee," with respect to Bob Marley's feel-good song title. The caffeine in coffee provides a natural jolt to your nervous system. A cup of coffee can be naturally refreshing, so it provides a pick-me-up that tastes heavenly and will give you that extra kick like listening to uplifting reggae music.

8 **BONE LOSS (Nourish your bones):** Just like losing your mojo, osteoporosis can be the devil's curse, too. The loss of bone density is often thought of an older person's disease—but it can strike at any age. Bone loss can happen for many reasons, including if you have a small, thin frame (like I do), a family history of

osteoporosis, are postmenopausal (like I am), are sedentary (as an author I am guilty), and eat a diet low in dairy products and other sources of calcium.

The Coffee Rx to Use: Drink a 8-ounce café au lait each day. Also, add a 12-ounce coffee smoothie with calcium-rich ice cream and low-fat milk in your diet regime regularly.

Why You'll Be Perked Up! Coffee paired with bone-boosting, calcium-rich milk can do your bones good. Calcium deficiency may also be connected with an increased risk for bone loss. Drinking black coffee with sugar, smoking, eating a poor diet, and not exercising will not beat bone loss just like a café au lait solo. It's the bone-boosting package that can help you to keep your bones strong. An extra bonus: Always add low-fat milk to coffee, the more the better.

9 **BRAIN DRAIN (Wake up your creative juices):** Feeling blah can drag you down and when you're dealing with "brain fog" it can be just as bothersome, especially if you're on the job and need to stay alert to get the job done. Coffee, a well-loved mind booster, is just the thing that can put your brain back in working order.

What Coffee Rx to Use: Order an 8-ounce or 12-ounce white coffee latte. It contains more caffeine than a regular latte—and that means you'll boost brain power. Go for a medium-blend coffee, which has more caffeine than a lighter or darker roast.

Why You'll Be Perked Up! Getting a buzz from caffeine works wonders. When a chemical in your brain, such as adenosine, hooks up with specific receptors, drowsiness sets in. But when caffeine comes to the rescue and mingles with the receptors your adrenal glands make adrenaline—and caffeine boosts dopamine to give you that feel-good caffeine fix.

10 **BULIMIA (Savor a day starter):** Nutrition plays a role in bone loss as it does in eating disorders. While you are imagining that you're overweight or have a fear that you will pack on the pounds, bulimia can wreak havoc on your health. Binging on unhealthful food—and purging—to maintain an ideal weight is a way of life for countless people, both women and men (all ages). Eating a nutrient-dense diet, exercising regularly, and finding a sense of

self and balance can help fight the imbalance—and coffee may come into play.

What Coffee Rx to Use: Each morning drink a 12-ounce cup of brewed medium-roast Colombian flavored coffee. Add low-fat milk to your taste.

Why You'll Be Perked Up! If you adopt a regular coffee habit in moderation, this low-cal beverage rich in antioxidants will also give you an energy boost to exercise. Not only will you boost your metabolism, but you'll burn calories when you get a move on. Also, this way you can eat healthful breakfast foods that'll lead into eating light and healthy all day long. The end result: You'll gain control of your diet and lifestyle and lose the roller-coaster ride of overeating and binging.

11 **BURNOUT (Grab a picker-upper):** Getting your diet back in balance can be your mission, but dealing with job or relationship burnout (when you just don't want to do it anymore) can be a problem, too. Coffee isn't a cure-all, but it can help you to enhance brainpower and physical energy so you can take a break and get back into the groove, especially when you are needed to get the job done whether you're done or not.

What Coffee Rx to Use: Opt to sip a 12-ounce café au lait (strong hot coffee with half hot milk) or your favorite flavored coffee with spices, including cinnamon and dark chocolate shavings.

Why You'll Be Perked Up! The idea of savoring a flavored coffee like hazelnut or French vanilla paired with a cinnamon stick and dark chocolate shavings will give your body a boost, mentally and physically. That means you may get the brainstorm to take a break—not just a coffee break. Yes, if you take a hiatus or at least get some R&R when you return to your life you'll be rejuvenated.

12 **CABIN FEVER (Get a feel-good jolt):** Burnout happens to all of us, sooner or later, but cabin fever may only hit those who live in a mountain town or region with erratic weather. Imagine being stuck in the house due to Mother Nature's wrath. It can drive you insane. The cure? Coffee.

What Coffee Rx to Use: Make an 8-ounce or 12-ounce café mocha and use dark chocolate with 70 percent cocoa content. Or try a dark chocolate coffee bar or truffles.

Why You'll Be Perked Up! Both dark chocolate and coffee contain feel-good compounds. Chocolate has got the endorphintheobromine to give you that lift that'll help stimulate your mind and body. A cup of fresh-brewed coffee or candy boasts caffeine and it will enhance mental and physical energy (it helps if you have a treadmill or free weights if you can't go outdoors) year-round.

Finding Your Zen

Sometimes, due to circumstances we cannot control, our lives are out of whack and we lose our balance. While we can't change certain events, we can change how we deal with potholes on our life's path. A tweak in our attitude can be helped with a bit of java, just as author Patricia Mote and her husband did:

It had been raining off and on for weeks; were we ever going to see the sun again? As well as slogging through the wet, we had both been working overtime to finish projects that were needed yesterday. Talk about tired; we had hardly been able to do more than grunt at one another. It was break time or we would break. Time for mindcation. No way could we physically leave town, but mentally, yes.

So I got out the Caribbean music, the rum and OJ, rubbed some chicken with my "Global Spice Rub," and transported us to the islands, any island. If we couldn't get on a sailboat this would have to do.

Global Spice Rub

❖ ❖ ❖

I call this global because the spices come from all over the world. The coffee makes this rub very special. Try the rub; it is also wonderful on grilled extra firm tofu or pork.

2 tablespoons chili powder
1 tablespoon unsweetened cocoa
2 tablespoons turbinado sugar
Dash cayenne
½ teaspoon smoked Spanish paprika

2 tablespoons very finely ground French Roast coffee
1 tablespoon sea salt
½ teaspoon cumin
½ teaspoon ground sumac

Mix all the rub ingredients together and then rub each piece of chicken with about 1 tablespoon of the rub. Grill for 10 minutes per inch of thickness.

13 **COLDS (Spice it up with liquid lightning):** Cabin fever does exist and it's a bear when you want to go outdoors but can't— much like catching a bad cold. One fall day on my birthday I caught a cold. First came the telltale scratchy sore throat, followed by sneezing and sniffling. I felt lousy and took to bed. The TV remote was in one hand and my companion animals surrounding me for comfort. The thing about getting sick is that you want to pamper yourself and resting is in order. You may think that doctor's orders would exclude a cup of coffee, but that's not necessarily so.

What Coffee Rx to Use: Take one aspirin and drink one 8-ounce cup of your favorite medium-roast coffee. Hold flavorings, sugar, and cream. Add 1 teaspoon of raw honey. Repeat two to three times each day.

Why You'll Be Perked Up! Since caffeine is used in aspirin and other pain relievers, it's not rocket science that if you take an aspirin paired with a hot or cold coffee (depending on the climate) it can help to lessen your misery—sooner rather than later.

There are dozens of antioxidants in both coffee and honey that can help fight a cold and bolster your immune system. The odds are the caffeine in coffee and flavor (if you drink a good cup of java) will make you feel better, mind, body, and spirit.

I'm not saying you'll be good to go and be ready to run a marathon, but chances are you'll enjoy that sabbatical a bit more, whether it is reading a book, watching a movie, or doing what you have to do. Read: Sometimes when we are coping with a cold, the dog(s) need to be walked, cat has to be fed, and other family members' needs must be met. Life goes on and coffee in moderation may be your best friend during a cold. A bonus: When a cold hits it's important to stay hydrated, and water is a big part of a cup of coffee, so don't count it out.

14 COUGHS (Sip the tickle away): Colds are pesky, but when a cough tailgates one, it's double trouble. Drinking coffee to help shake a cough isn't realistic, but a cup of this versatile beverage teamed with other home cures may be more helpful than you know.

What Coffee Rx to Use: Drink one cup of American medium roast once you begin coughing. Add 1 teaspoon of fresh lemon and 1 teaspoon of fresh, raw honey.

Why You'll Be Perked Up! Because coffee contains anti-inflammatory properties, it can help stave off chest aches from coughing. Lemon and honey will help coat your throat and soothe that tickle in your throat. Also, if you have a raspy voice it can help remedy that problem, too. This home cure is tried and tested by me. When I talk on the phone (and I do a lot), sometimes my voice gets too hoarse. This sweet coffee-lemon-honey cure helps keep my voice smoother.

15 DENTAL WOES (Enjoy a healthy mouth): Irregularity comes and goes, often due to a disrupted lifestyle, but keeping your teeth and gums healthy is a full-time gig no matter what's going on in your life. Tooth decay is not a fun experience, especially when your dentist gives you the diagnosis that can lead to feeling blue. Back in the 20th century cavities plagued more people, or so it seems. That doesn't mean adults, these days, are immune. And, of course, when we hear the dentist say, "You have a cavity," it can be a downer, due to anticipating the cost and drill. Coffee has the power to fight dental infections like cavities, plaque (the sticky stuff on your teeth from food), and the presence of bacteria in the gums. It also helps to control bleeding gums.

What Coffee Rx to Use: Opt to drink one or two 8-ounce cup(s) of coffee (especially instant) each day without sugar or flavorings to get the full benefit of its dental work.

Why You'll Be Perked Up! Coffee made from roasted coffee beans has antibacterial properties that work against certain microorganisms, including *Streptococcus mutans*, a major cause of dental cavities. Instant coffee had a somewhat higher level of inhibitory activity against *S. mutans*. Evidently, caffeine is not part of the antiadhesive properties of coffee solutions. Researchers suggested that trigonelline, a water-soluble compound in coffee that contributes to the aroma and flavor of the beverage, may be the key for coffee as an anticavity protector.[3]

16 **DEPRESSION (Lose the gloom and doom):** Now that the cough is under control, you may be one of the 10 percent of Americans experiencing a melancholy misery. No one is immune. The 21st century comes with a mixed bag of stressors, including from love problems or lack of love to money matters or no job.

What Coffee Remedy to Use: Try a 12-ounce cup of medium roast (City) or dark roast (Italian or French) two times each day. Better yet, make that organic java. Add milk and dark chocolate.

Why You'll Be Perked Up! There is light at the end of the dark tunnel for gloom and doom during tough times. Drinking a couple of cups of coffee daily can boost mood. Also, adding milk, a mineral that can calm nerves and muscles, plus dark chocolate, which contains tryptophan, can help lessen anxiety and stress (which often are linked to depression).

Hot Coffee May Keep Away a Superbug

Research shows that drinking a steaming hot cup of java may lessen developing MRSA (methicillin-resistant *Staphyloccocus aureus*) bacteria in your nose. That's right; your nose knows that there may be antimicrobial properties in coffee that may be linked to lowering the risk of carrying MRSA bacteria in your nasal passages.

Approximately 2.5 million people have MRSA inside their noses. In a study at the Medical University of South Carolina, Charleston, the more coffee (or tea) people drank, the lower their risk was for MRSA. The reason why hot coffee may be a preventative cure is because it contains compounds that may have antimicrobial properties that weaken the superbug. Despite the findings, the jury is still out, since antibiotics also have microbial properties but don't work wonders ridding people of MRSA.[4]

17 **DETOX YOUR BODY (Dump the toxins with a cup of mud):** Depression is right out depressing, and chances are you, like me, at one time or another have felt down. Well, our bodies can feel "depressed" if we pollute them with junk food, overindulge in unhealthy fare or alcohol. When you're body is polluted, that'll drag your spirit down, too. It doesn't have to be a spring detox—you can turn to cleansing your body any time of year. Total fasting is too taxing on the body, nutritionists agree, but a minifast is gentle and can do a body good. Eating fresh fruits and vegetables and drinking herbal teas, water, and coffee can be part of a healthful quickie minifast.

What Coffee Remedy to Use: Drink a 12-ounce cup of fresh-brewed medium roast (American or City) paired with 1 teaspoon each of unfiltered apple cider vinegar and raw honey.

Why You'll Be Perked Up! By drinking coffee a few times per day—in conjunction with produce, tea, and water—you can help detox your body in a variety of ways. First, coffee can help you eliminate toxins in your body. While you consume water-dense foods and beverages, you'll be energized with the help of java and more likely to get exercise, which can help you to sweat—another way to detox. If you follow this plan for one or two days, you'll feel more energized, lighter, and cleaner inside and outside. It will show in your face and body.

18 **DIARRHEA (Soothe your plumping):** Going to the bathroom more than you care to go—sometimes part of a detox fast—can be uncomfortable and an inconvenience. Blame it on a variety of reasons, from the stomach flu to traveling and having a bad reaction to food or water. You may think coffee would be the last thing to treat a bout of "Montezuma's Revenge," but maybe it's the first remedy to consider in an arsenal to fight back.

What Coffee Rx to Use: Try one 8-ounce cup of Colombian coffee with a fresh cinnamon stick one or two times per day.

Why You'll Be Perked Up! Coffee with its water content will help keep you hydrated. Plus, the feel-good caffeine will make you feel better rather than worse. The cinnamon is a known spice that is used for stomach troubles. Also, eating the BRAT diet—bananas, rice, applesauce, and toast—can be helpful, too, while you let the java spice beverage do its work.

19 **DIGESTION PROBLEMS (Soothe your stomach):** If coffee can be helpful for keeping you regular and dehydrated during a spell of the runs, it isn't to be avoided during a time of tummy woes. My suggesting you can treat irritable bowel syndrome (IBS: a spastic colon that has a mind of its own) with coffee may make you wonder: "Are you kidding?" but it can work for some people.

What Coffee Remedy to Use: Drink one 8-ounce cup of low-acid coffee with or without 1 tablespoon of manuka honey (less than 10 UMF). Or, if preferred, try adding fresh ginger in your coffee.

Why You'll Be Perked Up! Low-acid coffee is gentle on the stomach, but you still get the benefits of caffeine to give you a feel-good boost. Also, honey can help soothe an upset stomach, caused by the bacteria strain *Helicobacter pylori*. Honey can slow the growth of the bacteria.

When I was in my twenties, IBS haunted me, partly because of my diet and partly because of my stressful, erratic schedule. These days, following a regular lifestyle, eating a fiber-rich diet (whole grains, fruits, and vegetables), drinking bottled water and herbal tea, exercising to help keep me de-stressed, and drinking coffee every morning in moderation helps me stay regular and keep stomach woes at bay.

20 **DIZZINESS (Get balanced):** Feeling light-headed or dizzy can be linked to many causes, from prescription medications to hormonal changes, dehydration, high altitude, heat, and change in blood pressure. It's unsettling to not have your equilibrium, but if it's not a serious problem natural remedies can come to the rescue. I'm talking about getting sufficient water—and that includes a cup of java.

What Coffee Rx to Use: Drink one or two cups of flavored Colombian—flavored half decaf or decaf—each day along with breakfast starting in the morning and/or in the afternoon or after dinner.

Why You'll Be Perked Up! Coffee and its contents of water can help keep you both hydrated and alert. It's also essential to graze throughout the day to regulate your blood sugar levels so you will feel like a rock. If you don't eat or drink enough liquids, this can lead to low blood sugar and feeling light-headed or fainting can be the result. So, java and food are two ways to feel strong and steady.

21 **DRY MOUTH (Sip your mouth moist):** Feeling dizzy can be more unsettling than dry mouth, aka "Xerostomia," but that doesn't mean lack of saliva isn't bothersome. If your mouth sometimes gets dry, such as when you take medication, wet and warm coffee can come to the rescue to relieve your misery.

The Coffee Rx to Use: Try drinking one 8-ounce cup of cappuccino—a drink of coffee, milk, and chocolate. Repeat twice a day if needed.

Why You'll Be Perked Up! A mere five minutes of drinking 15.0 g of cappuccino coffee can increase the amount of saliva, decrease dry mouth, and improve the ability to speak, discovered researchers in Poland.[5]

22 **FATIGUE (Get a pick-me-up):** Dry mouth can be a drag, but if you're dragging your feet complaints may be more rather than

less. After all, we need energy to work and play and enjoy life. If fatigue is due to lack of shut-eye or burning the candle at both ends, coffee may come to your rescue.

The Coffee Rx to Use: Order a 16-ounce café mocha (with dark chocolate flavoring and dark chocolate shavings) at a coffee shop or make your own at home.

Why You'll Be Perked Up! It's a fact: Caffeine boosts your mental and physical energy. Dark chocolate contains theobromine, which like caffeine has a stimulating effect on the central nervous system. Anandamide, aka the "bliss chemical," occurs naturally in the brain and when released to our brain receptors can boost good feelings. Millions of people every day get a jump-start in the morning by drinking a cup of coffee (or two) to enjoy that jolt so they can get a move on.

23 **FLU (Shake the aches and pains):** Getting and staying bright eyed and energized is good, and life without aches and pains due to a quick onset of the dreaded flu is great. During the fall and winter the flu can hit you suddenly, and it's not fun to be out of commission, especially when life is calling for you to participate. But if the flu visits you there may be a way to say goodbye faster.

The Coffee Rx to Use: Try one 12-ounce cup of medium roast (for its antioxidants) and hold flavorings, cream, and sugar. Add lemon or orange slices and honey. Repeat in moderation as needed. Also, drink plenty of water, herbal tea, and fresh juices.

Why You'll Be Perked Up! Coffee is a super pick-me-up, which will give you the energy that'll help you to feel better. It contains the component quinic acid—and this is what gives coffee that sour acidic taste. It's a natural compound found in apples, peaches, and pears. It's also one of the primary ingredients in the Tamiflu formula—the stuff that people take when the flu hits home. Tamiflu is a pricey prescription medicine that is known for shortening flu symptoms. And remember, coffee also contains anti-inflammatory properties—key to fighting pain, which could be a godsend if you're fighting the flu. A bonus: Citrus is immune boosting and honey is antibacterial to help prevent a respiratory infection.

24 **GALLSTONES (Revamp your diet):** Did you know over-indulging in high-fat and cholesterol-rich food can lead to a gall-stone attack? Getting a gallstone stuck in the duct that leads from the gallbladder—where bile acids used for fat digestion are stored—to the upper intestine. Women are more at risk than men, perhaps due to hormones, and being overweight and smok-ing doesn't help, either. Age sometimes can be a factor and eat-ing too much rich food can be a trigger. But the word is, black coffee (not the high-fat flavored drinks) can be helpful to stave off the pain located in the right side of the chest below the breastbone and/or between the shoulder blades.

The Coffee Rx to Use: Incorporate coffee—black, regular-medium roast—in your diet every morning. Hold sugar, whole milk, creamers, and syrups.

Why You'll Be Perked Up! It is believed coffee may alter the metabolism of bile acids, which trigger the formation of the cho-lesterol crystals that become gallstones. Coffee also stimulates gallbladder contractions, which may curb stone formation.[6] It also gives you extra energy to stay physical, so you'll be more apt to keep your weight in check. Plus, a cup of antioxidant-rich cof-fee has less fat and calories than empty-nutrition high-fat fare or alcohol.

25 **GOUT (Wake up and enjoy your coffee):** Like gallstones, gout often occurs when you eat a high-fat diet and are carrying un-wanted extra pounds. It's made worse by eating liver, shellfish, and scallops.

The Coffee Rx to Use: Consider savoring a few 8-ounce cups of medium-roast flavored java on a daily basis.

Why You'll Be Perked Up! Boomer men at risk for gout should wake up and smell the coffee. B.C. researchers found the risk of gout was 40 percent lower for men who drank four to five cups a day than non–coffee drinkers. The news in today's *Journal of Rheumatology* shows this to be true.[7]

26 **HANGOVER (Say good-bye to the "ugh"):** Avoiding gout is probably easier than falling victim to a killer hangover. Paying the price of a headache after overindulgence in booze can and does

happen from celebrating or escaping woes. Then, your body has to deal with feeling terrible.

What Coffee Rx to Use: Try one 12-ounce cup of medium-roast coffee with 1 tablespoon of honey and an aspirin.

Why You'll Be Perked Up! Coffee contains caffeine, so if you team it with an aspirin it can work faster to help cure a headache. A cup of coffee paired with an over-the-counter anti-inflammatory painkiller may do the trick, blocking the headache compound culprit—acetate. Also, honey is rich in fructose and enzymes—which can boost metabolism of alcohol so you can shake that headache.

27 **HEADACHE (Stop the pain cold):** Hangovers are self-induced by overindulgence in alcohol, whereas headaches are triggered by a mixed bag of reasons. Ironically, caffeine—found in coffee—is a common trigger to headaches, but it can also help to make the pain go away.

What Coffee Rx to Use: One 12-ounce cup of coffee can help you reduce your suffering. A coffee with dark chocolate, such as a cappuccino or café mocha, can be helpful, too, due to its magnesium, which can help alleviate headaches. Also, keep your coffee intake steady and timely.

Why You'll Be Perked Up! The link between coffee and headaches is a tricky one. New York Headache Center's Alexander Mauskop, M.D., told me that when drunk infrequently in small amounts regular coffee (not decaf) can be helpful in treating tension headaches. "This is because caffeine has some pain-killing properties, gets to the brain quickly, and helps in the absorption of other medications," he explains. Ever notice it's an ingredient included in over-the-counter headache medications such as Excedrin and prescription drugs such as Fioricet? But note, if you're predisposed to having headaches, the limit is one cup a day, adds Dr. Mauskop.

Money Matters? Get a Boost from Joe

A sluggish economy can cause a lot of health ailments, from headaches and anxiety to depression and stress. The word is, people are cutting back, and purchasing a cup of pricey coffee in the morning is being tossed out along with going out to lunch.

But the good news is, you can still include coffee in your life and stay happy and healthy. Melanie Cox, a journalist in Pittsburgh, Pennsylvania, for one, isn't saying good-bye to java—she's thinking outside of the box to fit quality java into her daily grind each day:

Our family is on a tight budget, but my husband and I indulge in really good coffee. Our favorite roasters are Stumptown from Portland and Union Market's from Brooklyn. We order good gourmet beans online and get it shipped to us in Pittsburgh. We freeze it and use as needed. Our grinder is the basic Krups bullet (easy to use modest-priced grinder that makes a nice grind), but I have been envying the new Cuisinart grinder at work—you can turn the dial to fine, medium, or coarse, set the number of cups, and let it go automatically.

We brew about six cups in the morning and take it with us on our commute in those ceramic cups that look like coffee-shop paper cups with rubber sleeves. Too much coffee makes me a little jittery, but just the right amount makes me feel like a million bucks.

28 HOT FLASHES (**Nurse a cool cure**): Headaches to hot flashes (yes, I experienced my share) are a middle-aged woman's scourge. I admit that while I fell victim to hot flashes I also can say I learned what the the triggers were, including stress and hot beverages.

What Coffee Rx to Use: Make or buy a frappe (also called latte granite). Think iced Frappuccino at Starbucks. It's served cold: espresso, milk, sugar, and ice blended. You can ask for flavoring, like vanilla or chocolate. Or an iced cappuccino will suffice.

Why You'll Be Perked Up! A cold drink will refresh you and keep hot flashes at bay. Green tea has been praised by Japanese women, who do not experience hot flashes like we American women do. Iced coffee with antioxidant powers as well as feel-good caffeine just may be the new green tea for coffee lovers who go through the "pause" (and their men who stand by them).

29 **HYPOTENSION (Raise that blood pressure):** Hot flashes are uncomfortable, but hypotension (low blood pressure) can be more of a problem if it's an ongoing issue. If your BP reading is too low, symptoms of feeling light-headed, dizzy, or even faint may be part of the deal.

What Coffee Rx to Use: Drink one 8-ounce cup of organic medium-roast coffee, freshly brewed (not instant).

Why You'll Be Perked Up! The caffeine (which can vary from 85 to 135 milligrams) will boost your blood pressure just enough to prevent potentially dangerous symptoms. In the morning often blood pressure is low from a good night's rest. Sipping that morning cup of joe is a nice pick-me-up and can pick up those numbers right and put them in a nice and healthful comfort zone— 120/80 or a bit less. Organic will help relax your busy mind about unwanted pesticides. No kidding.

30 **IMMUNE SYSTEM (Get a daily immunity boost):** Hot flashes come and go, but then you end up getting a cold, flu, asthma, or allergies and even cancer—it can be linked to a weakened immune system. The immune system—that is, your body's defense system, made up of billions of white blood cells or "warriors" that are ready to destroy potential enemies—can protect you against illness, and coffee can help to bolster an immune system.

What Coffee Rx to Use: Drink two 8-ounce cups of medium roast coffee or honey lattes each day. Add a teaspoon of medicinal honey in a cup of immune-boosting tea for a double effect.

Why You'll Be Perked Up! Medium roast boasts antioxidants to help fight disease and keep your immune system strong. Because coffee contains caffeine it can give you energy to exercise, another way to keep your immunity up and resistance good to fight off the flu bug and other immunity monsters. And honey has antibacterial effects to sweeten and healthy up your coffee.

31 **INSOMNIA (Sleep like a baby):** If waking up to the fact that coffee is more than a jolt of caffeine surprises you, finding out that a cup of coffee won't disturb your sleep may be shocking. It's not recommended to drink several cups of coffee, but in moderation java junkies can get their fix of the antioxidant-rich, caffeinated beverage and get their seven to eight hours' nightly shut-eye, too.

    What Coffee Rx to Use: In the morning, savor one 6-ounce cup medium-roast coffee with milk or a honey latte.

    Why You'll Be Buzzed: More than a century ago, medical researchers discovered that caffeine can boost motor skills and reaction time while leaving sleep patterns alone. I don't need a study to prove that this supercompound (in moderation) does its job. During the busy day, I'll enjoy a cup of coffee in the A.M., to provide both mental and physical energy to work and walk the dogs, then swim. Sometimes, in the afternoon I'll sip another cup of brew to keep on working. Due to a full day of physical and mental tasks, coffee doesn't get in the way of sweet dreams.

32 **JET LAG (Perk up to a smooth postflight):** Jet lag happens when we disrupt our normal "circadian" rhythms that help us wake up in the morning and go to sleep at night. Drinking coffee helps counter the effects caused by jet lag and helps us to function normally by improving our ability to communicate and to boost our short-term memory. So, when we have to take a jet plane, can java juice help us get through the imbalance of our bodies and minds?

    Coffee Rx to Use: Drink small amounts (2-ounce or 4-ounce) of medium-roast brew on a regular basis during the day both at your new destination and also when you return home.

    Why You'll Be Perked Up! Caffeine, a primary ingredient in coffee, can help you to fight the jet lag blues, thanks to the hypothalamus gland, the main control center of the body clock in the brain, by shifting into a pattern that fits in with the time zone of your destination.[8]

33 **KIDNEY STONES (Chase away those bad boys):** Jet lag can feel like being in a sci-fi nightmare that won't end, but if you (or

someone you know) experiences the real world of kidney stones it's scary painful. A friend of mine was cursed by the stones and his tale of woe was unforgettable, from seeking professional help, to the treatments, and to follow-up at home care. It's enough to turn to coffee as a preventative measure.

The Coffee Rx to Use: Opt to drink one 12-ounce cup of medium or dark roast each morning.

Why You'll Be Perked Up! A steamy cup of coffee might be just what the doctor should order to help you lower your odds of getting kidney stones. Like alcohol (ever notice when people who drink beer have to go often?), caffeine in coffee waters down your urine and makes you go to the bathroom. That gives kidney stones less of a chance to develop. But don't ignore decaf, because researchers believe that something other than caffeine is the helper.[9]

34 **LOW LIBIDO (Finding your groove, again):** Speaking of woes below the belt, at any age your sex drive may wax and wane due to stress, hormones, work, kids, poor communication, or maybe you're just not that into him or her. Can coffee boost sex drive? The answer to this question is a tricky one. Personally, I can attest that caffeine can give me a physical and mental lift—and that it can tweak the mind and maneuver thoughts to romance. What's more, if you and you know who are tired, a cup of joe may be all you two need. Take the quality time to drink a comforting cup of coffee and ignite intimacy and that may be all that you need to nudge the love bug into the throes of passion.

What Coffee Rx to Use: Drink one 12-ounce cup of your favorite flavored Colombian coffee (with or without a shot of alcohol) and dark chocolate.

Why You'll Be Perked Up! Dark chocolate and alcohol both have been touted for their merits of enhancing the sex drive. Alcohol can reduce inhibitions and help you to relax. Dark chocolate contains compounds that induce feel-good endorphins (just like after exercise or lovemaking).

If your libido makes a hit you can give credit to java and its companions. Or if you and your partner don't make love, the odds are you'll connect on a mental level and a rain check could be in order with a promise of lovemaking. Either way, it's a win-

win situation. And, if nothing happens at least coffee and its healthful compounds will help keep you well and provide you with a sense of well-being.

Just ask author Patricia Mote, a resident of Annapolis, Maryland. She knows too well how java heats things up, especially if you make the most of your situation:

The snow had started in the middle of the night and by dawn was already four feet deep; a real Sierra snowfall. We were snuggled in our down comforters watching, not wanting to break the magnificent silence. But one thing seemed certain; this was a morning for a real New Orleans style Café au Lait.

Per drink: ¾ cup dark roast coffee with chicory; ½ cup scalded milk. Pour the coffee and milk together into a large cup. Or do as the French do and pour it into a bowl so large you have to surround it with two hands. All the better to inhale the delicious aroma as I settled back into the comforters with my honey. Now if we only had some beignets! (See chapter 18, "Here Comes the Coffee.")

Coffee Chat on the Silver Screen

Speaking of aphrodisiacs, a cup of cappuccino and foreplay go back centuries. Think of films and real-life people who go to bistros and coffee shops to meet, sit, and enjoy a titillating conversation—a meeting of the minds.

Coffee, whether it's espresso or a latte, gives you a caffeine buzz that can stimulate both your mind and body, thus feel good, and talking to someone you care about can be romantic.

Of course, coffee scenes on the big screen aren't always the scenes of great lovers, but they can end up that way. *You've Got Mail,* for instance, shows Tom Hanks and Meg Ryan meeting at a coffeehouse. The one-on-one conversation turns out to be anything but what a budding relationship should be, but the witty banter is unforgettable and the end result was a happy ending.

In the cult film *Pulp Fiction,* the coffee shop scenes show a lot of heat but not necessarily the type of romance one dreams about. Not to forget *Dante's Peak*. Even during the ongoing volcanic eruption, Linda Hamilton's character (a mayor who runs a coffee shop) tries to stall a loving moment with a cup of coffee.

And, moving on from love to work, *The Devil Wears Prada* is a grueling wake-up call for anyone who has fetched a cup of java for a boss, like loyal Anne Hathaway's character does. While working her way through the mean streets of New York, she retrieves Starbucks coffee to deliver to the "devil" in order to keep her job.

And, chatting about coffee on the big screen, I cannot forget *Vanished*, a film that shows to what lengths a lover will go to reconnect with a lost lover—even if it entails drinking drug-spiked coffee from a thermos to find out what happened to the one who got away.

35 **MOODINESS (Brew your balance):** Whether you're solo or in a relationship, mood swings can hit anytime at home or work. Coffee may be just what you need to feel that loving feeling. Coffee is not a cure-all fix to the ebb and flow of life's lemons that get tossed our way—but a morning with the mood-boosting beverage does seem to uplift the mind and spirit.

What Coffee Rx to Use: Brew a fresh 8-ounce cup (or two) of medium or dark Colombian roast coffee and stay clear of adding sugar or syrups.

Why You'll Be Perked Up! That jolt of caffeinated coffee with your breakfast can put you in a good mood and much more. Scientists at the University of Wales College of Cardiff in the UK discovered people given caffeine not only do better performing tasks that use memory and logical reasoning but also reported greater alertness and feelings of well-being.[10]

36 **MUSCLE CRAMPS (Shake that pain):** Mood swings can make you feel like you're on an amusement park ride, but muscle cramps can make you wish you didn't have to ride out the pain. Muscle cramps can occur in many places on your body, and if you have a natural cure available it would be senseless not to try it for potential relief without side effects.

What Coffee Rx to Use: One 8-ounce cup of regular coffee (try a medium roast with citrus slices for its anti-inflammatory properties) upon enduring a muscle cramp or if you sense you may get one due to exercise or other factors. Or try a latte, because milk can alleviate muscle tension. Repeat as needed in moderation.

Why You'll Be Perked Up! The word is caffeine relieves muscle pain by blocking the activity of a chemical, called adenosine, that is released due to inflammatory response to injury. This chemical is responsible for the pain in body cells.[11]

37 **PINKEYE (Nurse it with java):** Muscle cramps can pay you an untimely visit and hurt a lot, but pinkeye can hurt and look painful, too. Pinkeye or conjunctivitis is an inflammation of the membrane covering the surface of your eyeball. It can be caused by bacteria, viruses, or allergens. Whatever the reason, discharge, redness, and pain are the end result. But can coffee help?

What Coffee Rx to Use: Try a dash of regular coffee grounds boiled in water until you have a dark solution. Cool. Put a small amount of the solution on the infected eye. Rinse.

Why You'll Be Perked Up! The coffee cure for pinkeye is available, easy to use, and inexpensive. This solution is a folk remedy that may or may not work. If you're out in the wilderness or another place without a doctor it could prove to be Plan B. However, if you're home and your eye infection is looking more serious than not, consult with a physician and hold the coffee.

38 **PMS (Chase the crankies and cravings):** Pinkeye can be pesky like premenstrual syndrome (PMS). I remember docs told me to stay clear of caffeine when I was suffering from PMS, but that was easier said than done. Often during the week of PMS, fatigue hits. Not to forget bloat and the blues. I ignored doctors' orders and followed my cravings. Coffee and chocolate helped me to cope.

What Coffee Rx to Use: Try a 12-ounce cup of mocha latte or a mocha shake.

Why You'll Be Perked Up! Both coffee and chocolate will give you an energy boost and boost well-being. Also, since coffee can help to suppress your appetite, eating sweets with too many calories and not enough nutrients won't be so tempting. A moderate jolt from java can help get you motivated to get moving and engage in calorie-burning aerobic activities (or lovemaking). Getting physical can ignite feel-good endorphins that help to lessen PMS cramps and similar symptoms from menstrual periods, too, because it helps the blood flow.

39 **POOR HANDWRITING (Sweeten up your penmanship):** Perhaps messy writing isn't a pain, but it can be fatal. When a pro, perhaps even you, writes something that is unreadable and affects someone's life, such as a vet prescribing your prized pooch a medication or a doctor giving you a prescription and you end up getting a med for a canine that's scary. But coffee may be the cure to clear up those illegible letters, words, and numbers that require a large, round magnifying glass and patience.

What Coffee Rx to Use: Drink one 12-ounce cup of medium roast or mocha. Once finished, you should be ready to write. Repeat as needed, but moderation is recommended.

Why You'll Be Perked Up! Caffeine, the ingredient found in regular coffee (both brewed and instant), may be the ingredient to help you have more fluent movements and write more quickly, too. One study from Germany found that caffeine can produce improvements in handwriting.[12]

40 **ROUGH SKIN (Wake up to a smooth body):** Writing clearer, faster, and better is one thing, but dealing with skin that is dry can be a different type of burden. Soft and glowing skin is great to have and not too difficult to achieve if you spend some time to stave off the culprits and turn to helpers, like coffee used externally.

What Coffee Rx to Use: Each day when you bathe, apply coffee grounds with olive oil or a store-bought product on your skin from neck to toe. (Flip to chapter 14, "The Beauty of Coffee," and discover all the reasons why this superfood can be your skin's best friend.)

Why You'll Be Perked Up! Coffee grounds have an abrasive effect, thanks to its texture and antioxidants that can help smooth rough skin and soften it and stave off inflammation of reddened skin. The end result: a nice, youthful glow and skin that feels nicer to touch. It helps to stay out of the sun and use sunscreen, wear clothing that screens your skin, use a humidifier if you live in a region with low humidity, and drink plenty of fluids—that includes coffee in moderation.

41 **SEASONAL AFFECTIVE DISORDER (Warm up and feel happy):** Shynesss isn't fun, but winter blues or seasonal affective disorder (SAD) during the cold, winter months may feel worse and lasts longer. Symptoms include weight gain, depression, lethargy, and loss of libido. What possibly could make you feel better if winter discontent hits you? Coffee can and does come to the rescue.

What Coffee Rx to Use: One 12-ounce Americano or cappuccino. Repeat as needed.

Why You'll Be Perked Up! First, the flavor of these coffee drinks will make you feel better and warm you up. Then, the caffeine fix will kick in and that's going to blast the winter blues away. You'll be ready to go shovel snow and/or go to work or play. Also, because caffeine can rev up your metabolism and give you energy, you'll burn off calories. Once you get a move on and are feeling better, the odds are your sex drive may pay you a visit during days and nights, especially if you enjoy a cup of java with that someone special and savor the highlights of winter: from enjoying a picturesque snowfall to cuddling up by a warm fireplace.

42 **SOCIAL ANXIETY (Perk up and enjoy):** Speaking of handwriting and skin, as an author I have frequented book lectures/signings—social gatherings. The truth of the matter is, I am an introvert. I prefer to work solo, amid a calm, human-free environment in the mountains amid my creature comforts—two dogs and a cat. Public speaking in person at a bookstore or on airwaves used to bother me, the shy girl.

Many book lecture/signings ago, I sat in a chair at a Barnes & Noble bookstore. I invited a guest speaker to keep the limelight off me. At first, I thought it was a good idea, because dozens of people arrived. Then, the store manager introduced me, the author, and handed me the microphone. I felt my face turn bright red as I saw people, lots of people, gathering to hear me speak. I got through the limelight experience and now I turn to the coffee cure before talking to an audience.

What Coffee Rx to Use: Brew one 8-ounce cup of medium roast—regular or honey latte. Add one fourth-cup milk. Hold the sugar.

Why You'll Be Perked Up! Coffee can give you a pick-me-up, socializing nudge—even if you've got a touch of social anxiety. Some folks who get shyness, like me, emphasize that the amount of coffee you drink matters. If you face social anxiety, lessen your intake of regular coffee and add milk. Or try decaffeinated coffee, which contains very little caffeine.

43 **SUMMER SAD (Boost your spirit):** Winter blues are depressing, but so is summertime—for some people. Imagine this scenario: The sky is blue, the sun is shining, couples, fit and lean, are outdoors participating in fun activities. But if you're single, introverted, you may find yourself irritable and fed up with longer days and too many people, especially if you live in a tourist town. The fact is, you may have Summer SAD. But don't despair, because coffee can be helpful.

What Coffee Rx to Use: Try a 12-ounce iced honey latte or latte. Repeat as needed.

Why You'll Be Buzzed: People with SAD often have low levels of serotonin (a compound found in honey and milk), a brain chemical believed to be involved in modulating mood and appetite. By sipping a mug or two of coffee with plenty of tryptophan-rich foods such as milk sweetened with honey you can boost levels of serotonin.

44 **SINUSITIS (Inhale the steamy aroma):** Summertime blues are dreadful (and sometimes I can fall into this malady), but sinus woes can be miserable, too. Welcome a killer headache between the eyes, sneezing, sniffling, congestion, and worse if it turns into a sinus infection. Cold weather compounded with lack of humidity and high altitude combined with central house heating (or air-conditioning) can exasperate your symptoms or trigger a sinus flare-up.

What Coffee Rx to Use: Opt for a 12-ounce cup of regular roast (medium or dark) with 2 tablespoons of honey and a dash of cinnamon. Repeat as needed.

Why You'll Be Perked Up! The sweet taste of honey and hot coffee spiked with spices (such as cinnamon) is just the combo to help clear your sinuses. Drinking water, which coffee does contain, also helps to loosen up mucus.

45 SLEEP DEPRIVATION (Wake up and smell the coffee): Sinusitis flare-ups are a challenge, but lack of shut-eye can affect your persona to the point of no return or fantasizing about boarding a shuttle to the next planet. The reasons for lack of sleep are varied, and most people will fall victim to sleep deprivation in their life, reveals research at the National Sleep Foundation. The thing is, sometimes we don't have a choice of sleeping like a lion and we must stay up.

What Coffee Rx to Use: Drink small amounts of medium roast throughout the day. To alleviate boredom, try different roasts (medium has the most caffeine) and don't hesitate to add real dark chocolate shavings in a café mocha (another eye-opener with its variety of feel-good compounds).

Why You'll Be Buzzed: Coffee can be your best friend if you're counting on something to help you stay awake through the day or night. Harvard medical researchers discovered that low-dose repeated caffeine used for circadian-phrase-dependent performance degradation driving extended wakefulness. In other words, coffee can help you get through the day or night.[13]

46 SLUGGISH SPORTS PERFORMANCE (Get a move on): If you're tired, you won't feel like running a marathon or doing much of anything that requires physical exertion. These days, year-round before I swim at noon I have a 12-ounce cup of coffee in my system. Not only does it help curb my appetite in the morning (I prefer a Continental breakfast, which is more in vogue than a huge meal fit for a king), but it also helps give me energy to enjoy my lap swimming.

What Coffee Rx to Use: A 12-ounce cup of mocha.

Why You'll Be Perked Up! Medical researchers and athletes are all too familiar with the energetic buzz linked to coffee. And yes, brewed coffee contains caffeine (approximately 85 milligrams per 8-ounce mug), much more than chocolate (1 ounce of semi-sweet dark chocolate contains about 20 milligrams of caffeine). I can vouch that coffee can boost your drive, endurance, and performance. Remember, moderation.

47 **STRESS (Escape tense times):** It's easier to beat a sluggish feeling than high stress, which can be triggered by pressure on the job, at home conflicts with family, friends, or neighbors, or natural events that cannot be controlled. The key to chilling is learning how to go with the flow. Finding natural, comforting ways—like coffee—to help you cope with circumstances beyond your control can help you take control of your composure and stay cool.

The Coffee Rx to Use: Try one 12-ounce honey latte or latte or your favorite flavored coffee, such as blueberry crumble or hazelnut. Repeat twice daily.

Why You'll Be Perked Up! Coffee can help you to feel alert and enhance your sense of well-being despite chaos. Milk can help you to de-stress because it's a calming mineral. If you team this beverage with fresh fruit to get antistress C vitamins you can chill during life's daily stressors.

48 **WATER RETENTION (Blast the bloat):** If you're stressed out it wouldn't be a surprise if your tummy is bloated, too. Bloating can hit when you're upset, are PMS-ing and retaining water, during the "pause" thanks to shifting hormones, and even when you're eating the wrong foods. Not only is bloat frustrating when your stomach is too puffy to wear your skinny jeans or favorite dress, but it's also often uncomfortable.

What Coffee Rx to Use: Try an 8-ounce cup or two of black medium roast with a slice or two of lemon. Drink a glass of water after for a double effect. Also, pair a cup of coffee with a piece of fresh water-dense fruit.

Why You'll Be Perked Up! Drinking bloat-busting lemony coffee, a natural diuretic because of its caffeine, citrus, and water content, will help alleviate pesky water retention that causes bloating. Plus, the potassium in fruit can help counteract unwanted sodium and bloat, too.

49 **WEIGHT GAIN (Put on healthy pounds):** So if coffee can help you dump from water weight to unwanted pounds and body fat,

how in the Coffee World can the beans help you to add weight? They can. The magical beans combined with additives in coffee beverages to coffee food pairings can help to add pounds if that's what you want to do. Sometimes, after getting sick, such as a flu bug, or if you lose a loved one or go through emotional turmoil due to stressors in life, eating may be the last thing on your mind.

What Coffee Rx to Use: Make a 12-ounce homemade coffee shake with premium coffee ice cream, brewed coffee, fresh fruit, whole milk, wheat germ, and ice cubes. Top with whipped cream and dark chocolate shavings. Pair with a slice of coffee cake. Repeat twice a day. Or try an *affogato* (espresso over vanilla ice cream) with a dollop or two of whipped cream.

Why You'll Be Perked Up! If you're trying to put on unwanted lost weight, it's best to drink coffee beverages with all-natural additives. There are all-natural coffee creamers and flavored syrups and powders (with added nutrients) and real whipped cream. Also, portion size comes into play. Rather than a 6-ounce or 8-ounce cup of joe, make a large coffee drink. Keep it natural and eat healthful food, including healthful fatty foods that go with coffee beverages, such as dark chocolate, chopped nuts, and whole milk.

50 **UNIVERSAL EMERGENCY AID** (Savor the buzz grounds): Wanting to pack on pounds may seem like an ER time if you're looking a bit thin. Still, a real emergency can rock your boat. Earthquakes, tornadoes, blizzards, and wildfires, to name just a few, can make it seem like your world has ended as you once knew it. Before or after, a cup of coffee may seem like a godsend to help you feel normal and hang in there.

What Coffee Rx to Use: Opt for a 12-ounce cup of instant coffee (flavored is a good choice).

Why You'll Be Perked Up! After enduring the 7.1 World Series earthquake back in 1989, I, like countless others in the San Francisco Bay Area, was stricken by aftershocks. Hesitant to brew a cup of coffee, I found it was quicker to make a cup of instant coffee (a pod coffeemaker is also a good idea to have for emergencies) and be done with it. The coffee was comforting and kept me awake as I kept on top of what the latest news was and tried to stay calm but prepared.

Smart Start Milkshake

❖ ❖ ❖

1 cup brewed coffee, cold
  or at room temperature
½ cup low-fat (1 percent)
  milk (substitute low-carb
  milk)
½ teaspoon peppermint
  extract

1 cup chocolate ice
  cream, slightly softened
  (substitute low-carb
  ice cream)
1 packet Splenda

Place all ingredients in a blender container. Cover, and blend on high speed for 1 minute, or until smooth. Pour into 2 tall glasses. Serve immediately. Makes two 12-ounce servings.

(*Courtesy:* Coffee Science Source.)

A CUP FULL OF PERKS

If it doesn't specify which form or variety of coffee to use, go ahead and use your coffee of choice—medium or dark roast is recommended for best results.

Ailment or Process	Coffee	What It May Do
Agorophobia	Medium roast, half decaf with milk	Lessen the phobia
Allergies	Dark roast with honey	Boost blood cells
Anxiety	Regular half decaf café au lait or latte	Soothe frazzled nerves
Asthma	Medium or dark roast	Relieve sneezing, congestion

Ailment or Process	Coffee	What It May Do
Attention Deficit Disorder	Medium roast	Aid in concentration
Baldness	Irish coffee, medium roast	Aid in hair growth
Blahs	Cappuccino or café au lait	Boost spirit
Bone loss	Café au lait, coffee smoothie	Strengthen bones
Brain drain	White coffee latte	Enhance mind
Bulimia	Medium roast, flavored Colombian	Provide nourishment
Burnout	Café au lait with spices	Aid in motivation
Cabin fever	Café mocha	Provide energy
Colds	Medium roast with honey	Help healing
Cough	Medium roast with honey and lemon	Soothe tickle
Dental woes	Instant coffee	Prevent cavities, gum problems
Depression	Medium or dark roast with chocolate	Uplift spirit
Detoxification	Medium roast with apple cider vinegar, honey	Cleanse body toxins
Diarrhea	Colombian roast with cinnamon	Help regulation

Ailment or Process	Coffee	What It May Do
Digestive problems	Low-acid coffee with honey and ginger	Soothe stomach upset
Dizziness	Flavored Colombian, half decaf, decaf	Hydrate and calm you
Dry mouth	Cappuccinio	Aid in saliva production
Fatigue	Café mocha	Boost energy
Flu	Medium roast with honey and citrus	Speed recovery
Gallstones	Medium roast, black	Prevent gallstones
Gout	Medium roast	Lower risk of gout
Hangover	Medium roast with aspirin	Speed recovery
Headache	Cappuccino or cafe mocha	Relieve pain
Hot flashes	Iced coffee	Alleviate the discomfort
Hypotension	Organic medium roast	Keep blood pressure normal
Immunity problems	Medium roast	Bolster immune system
Insomnia	Medium roast, honey latte	Induce good sleep
Jet lag	Medium roast	Normalize body and mind
Kidney stones	Medium roast	Lower risk
Low libido	Flavored Colombian roast (with a shot of alcohol)	Boosts sex drive

Ailment or Process	Coffee	What It May Do
Moodiness	Medium or dark roast	Uplift spirit
Muscle cramps	Latte or medium roast	Rid pain
Pinkeye	Regular roast	Lessen inflammation
PMS	Mocha latte or mocha shake	Lessen cramps, crankies
Poor handwriting	Medium roast, mocha	Improve penmanship
Rough skin	Coffee grounds	Smooth body
Seasonal Affective Disorder	Cappuccino or Americano	Boost mood, energy, lessen simple carb cravings
Sinusitis	Medium or dark roast with honey	Relieve stuffed-up nasal passages
Sleep deprivation	Medium roast	Help rejuvenate your mind and body
Sluggish sports performance	Medium roast, mocha, frappe	Energize stamina
Social anxiety	Medium roast, honey latte	Lessen inhibitions
Stress	Honey latte, flavored coffee	Calm nervous system
Summer SAD	Iced coffee, honey latte	Improve mood
Water retention	Medium roast	Help get rid of bloat
Weight gain	*Affogato*, coffee shake	Aid in adding pounds
Universal emergency	Instant coffee	Act as cure-all

In part 7, "Future Coffee," you'll wake up to the ongoing buzz about coffee—all types—that continues to percolate 24/7 in homes, offices, hospitals, coffeehouses and bistros, and restaurants, in America and around the globe, thanks to its versatile, natural uses in the home.

PART 7

FUTURE COFFEE

CHAPTER 13

Coffee Craze: Grounds for the Household

Coffee is real good when you drink it, it gives you time to think. It's a lot more than just a drink; it's something happening. . . . It gives you time, but not actual hours or minutes, but a chance to be, like yourself, and have a second cup.

—Gertrude Stein[1]

Like a full-grown coffee tree yielding beans, I started producing for local and national magazines and newspapers. I blossomed into a full-time journalist (often out in the field). Grabbing a coffee "with legs" or "on a leash" (to go, with handles) played a role both on the road and at the keyboard. Coffee—with its caffeine promise to boost brainpower—definitely was my trustworthy assistant, especially when meeting deadlines.

Living on the peninsula in the San Francisco Bay Area, an architect enduring a divorce and I bonded and became good friends—the kind that complain and get each other's challenges in the cruel world. One morning, before 7:00 A.M., I'd grabbed my article "15 Fat-fighting Foods" for *Woman's World* magazine that I completed during an all-nighter of research and rewrites. With my on-the-go Brittany, Dylan, I knocked on the back door (much like Ethel Mertz in an *I Love Lucy* episode) of Mr. Architect and was invited to pour a cup of freshly ground and brewed coffee. He also had the convenience of a fax machine (this was the nineties) and a dog pal for my canine. After half a cup of his strong brew I'd be wide awake.

In the evening after we both had put in a hard day's work, I'd go to his bungalow to relax. We'd kick back in the living room surrounded by an outdoor flower garden, overstuffed couches, a fireplace, and snuggled with our dogs, my Brittany Dylan and his Border collie, Daisy. And the refuge was enhanced by the bean juice as we sipped coffee for comfort and conversation, sharing chocolate bars and popcorn. It was utopia for two starving artists who enjoyed a minimalist's life.

In this chapter, I will show you that while comforting coffee is used as a superhealthful beverage to stay up and wake up, it's also making a splash in the United States and around the world for its versatile uses indoors and outdoors, too.

THE COFFEE CRAZE

The coffee phenomenon continues to soar around the world in the 21st century. Coffee consumption is strong and steady. The 2011 National Coffee Drinking Trends poll suggests a solid footing for future growth.

Take a look at these sobering statistics, straight from the 2011 National Coffee Drinking Trends Study.

- 40 percent of 18- to 24-year-olds drink coffee daily, up from 31 percent in 2010.
- 54 percent of adults age 25 to 39 said they drink coffee daily, up from 44 percent in 2010.
- These figures aligned with findings that 29 percent of those 18 to 39 felt better about their financial situation than last year, while other age groups did not.
- Gourmet coffee continues to be a significant portion (37 percent) of total coffee consumed, indicating that consumers want to maintain coffee quality despite the uncertain economy.

At Home Market

- 86 percent of coffee consumers enjoyed their beverage at home compared to 24 percent who drink out of the home, on par with 2010 findings. (Note that these figures include those who drink coffee both at home and away.)
- Penetration is growing in the single-serve arena at an average of 1 percent per year, and 35 percent of those with a pod system acquired it in the past six months. Purchasers of the pod system are now more likely to use it to replace their current brewer. There is an increased awareness of single-cup systems, with 45 percent who think the systems are excellent or very good in 2011, compared to 26 percent in 2007.

(*Courtesy*: NCA Market Research.)

WIDESPREAD COFFEE APPEAL

It's no surprise that coffee is a household commodity in the kitchen for people in the United States or that its versatile uses are praised around the globe, too. The chart below shows about 95 percent of the world's coffee production in the 21st century. Vietnam, for one, has doubled its production in the past decade and now produces more than Colombia, although its coffees compete with major coffee exporters such as Brazil, Colombia, and Indonesia. About a dozen countries have a significant share of the lucrative gourmet market. Here, take a look at countries (ranking in producing the most bags per year) making coffee for you.

Coffee Country	Typical Harvest Months
Brazil	April–September
Vietnam	N/A
Colombia	November–January and April–June
Indonesia	Varies
India	N/A
Mexico	October–December

Coffee Country	Typical Harvest Months
Mexico	October–December
Guatemala	October–December
Ethiopia	August–January
Côte d'Ivoire	N/A
Uganda	September–December
Honduras	December–February
Peru	N/A
Costa Rica	December–February

(*Courtesy:* Zecuppa Coffee.)

Coffeemania Time ... Did You Know?

1. Coffee shops make up the fastest-growing part of the restaurant business, checking in with a 7 percent annual growth rate.
2. World coffee production is estimated at 100 to 120 million bags per year.
3. Fourteen billion espresso coffees are consumed each year in Italy, reaching over 200,000 coffee bars, and still growing.
4. Americans consume 400 million cups of coffee per day, or equivalent to 146 billion cups of coffee per year, making the United States the leading consumer of coffee in the world.
5. Japan ranks number three in the world for consumption.
6. Coffee represents 75 percent of all the caffeine in the United States.
7. Café bars average sales of 230 cups a day.

(*Courtesy:* Coffee-Statistics.com.)

HEALING YOUR HOME ROOM BY ROOM

Drinking coffee for its healing powers is healing, but did you know that you can use coffee for healing your personal environment, too? Welcome to the world of coffee uses in the home, another perk of the coffee tree. Before I entered Coffee World, I didn't know coffee grounds were eco-friendly and something to use. I assumed the dark brown gritty grounds were something that my food-loving dog duo and cat who thinks he's a dog shouldn't get into and I'd put them into the garbage ASAP to avoid vet ER phone calls and visits. But now I know that while grounds aren't animal friendly they can be home friendly. Bless the little dark coffee grounds for their multi-purpose uses indoors and outdoors.

Kitchen

Use an Abrasive Cleaner: Use grounds as a scouring agent to tackle any greasy or dirty surface. It also can get rid of pungent odors from pans and your hands.

Go for a Deodorizing Buzz: Dry coffee ground (not soggy used ones) placed on a cookie sheet and put in an open container in your fridge or freezer can be an instant way to help absorb odors. Also, fill a sachet with dried grounds paired with cinnamon sticks and whole cloves and place it in closed drawers (baby and pet proof).

Living Room/Dining Room/Bedroom

Furniture Concealer: Coffee grounds can do away with smells and unsightly scratches on furniture, too. Steep grounds and apply the dark brew to wood furniture with a cloth. I tried this household treatment on an antique dark chest in my bedroom and it worked. I thought, "If coffee stains cups, coffeepots, and teeth, it has to work on brown furniture." And it did just that. Flavored coffees provide a nice aroma, unlike commercial types with strong, undesirable scents.

Fireplace Dust Buster: Ever notice that when you clean out the ashes from the fireplace dust gets in your eyes and nose? You can control the dust by using wet coffee grounds on the cool ashes because they keep the dust down and not in the air. Note to self: Try to see if this method works.

Bathroom

Ant Repellent: In the mountains I don't see ants, but in the city I did. And if they weren't in the kitchen they took over the bathroom, especially around water. Rather than using a chemical spray, try using coffee grounds on the area thirsty ants go to. (Be sure kids, cats, and dogs are not around as the natural anteater does its job.)

Outdoors

Plant Fertilizer: Plants that like acidic soils will like your coffee grounds. Use grounds on the top layer of soil, or mix them with potting soil before planting. I started dumping coffee grounds on the aspens in the front yard. It could have been the late-summer rain and/or the green grounds that helped the trees perk up.

Compost: Grounds not only feed your plants and trees, but they can feed your compost bin (if you have one) also. Simply add compost piles to increase nitrogen balance. Coffee filters and tea bags (yes, I have both, especially if my youngest Brittany doesn't scarf down the chamomile tea bags) will also break down fast during composting. I still don't do the compost dance, but it's on my list of to-do changes and coffee grounds and filters will be included. I continue to sprinkle grounds on one wilted aspen in the front yard, but so far it's not showing signs of being a coffee lover. . . .

Insect Repellent: But tossing coffee grounds on the deck, dirt, or sidewalks may have a faster effect. Again, it's a risk to do this if you have indoor/outdoor dogs or cats, because you don't want a sequel of the Ethiopian goat herder's dancing goats.

> ### Kingdom of Coffee
> ### (First Source, Kaffa, Ethiopia)
>
> We learned about the "birds and beans"
> From folks when we were growing up.
> How birds atwitter sometimes mean
> They've found a source to fill our cup.

If you need coffee night and day,
    You're ready for a coffee break;
A caffeine fiend, some people say,
    Can even keep his friends awake.

The Muslims first from Africa
    Made use of these most hallowed grounds.
Eventually America
    Found coffee needs right here abound.

I like a lot of latte some,
    But Javanese is just the thing
To make my mind and muscles hum
    And help my early mornings sing.

The "wine of bean," the Turks proclaim,
    In coffeehouses or cafés,
Where coffee culture earned its fame—
    Not Starbucks where we sing its praise.

A cuppa joe or mellow brew
    Around the world is what we need
To give both friends and foes a view
    Of happy times where we succeed.

—Jim Berkland, geologist
Glen Ellen, California

COFFEE CANDLES DELIGHT

Fall and winter are the perfect times to light up your home with sensual warmth—from a cup of coffee paired with the sweet scent of coffee candles. Naturally fragrant candles, scented with blends or aromatic extractions of coffee flavors, provide comfort to any room in the home.

Coffee candles made with different aromas such as amaretto coffee, café au lait, café mocha, cappuccino, and Irish cream can provide a mellow, earthy mood. I got creative and tried café mocha for the kitchen, cappuccino for the dining room/living room or study, and amaretto coffee for the bedroom or bathroom. The scent lingers like that of a batch of mocha brownies.

Versatile coffee candles can be used year-round, too. In the summertime, Lake Tahoe does have its chilly nights when the temperature can plummet to the thirties. Nothing is more comforting than to make a fire in the fireplace and to light a coffee candle. Add fresh-brewed coffee and home-baked cinnamon rolls to achieve an even more inviting vibe.

One summer day during a thunderstorm, I lit a large soy Hazelnut Coffee candle in my bathroom. It had a rich, full-bodied aroma accompanied by the appeal of roasted European hazelnuts and a touch of cream. The wood wick was something new to me. It crackled like the fires I make in my rustic rock fireplace during the wintertime. It was a soothing touch while I finished sipping a fresh cup of Chocolate Raspberry flavored coffee. I was inspired and piled fresh dark coffee brown towels on the countertop, next to a thick white robe (the kind I wore at a hotel in San Francisco). These little things—including the aroma of a coffee candle—can make any day, like that one, extraordinary and feed your mind, body, and spirit.

COFFEE SPILLS ON YOUR STUFF

Coffee candles and a cuppa java can be heavenly, but coffee stains are an eyesore, especially on light-colored curtains, tablecloths, or clothes. Try white vinegar, but nix apple cider or red wine vinegars. Mix 1/2 cup white distilled vinegar and 1 cup of cold water in a container. Use a paper towel (not colored ones) and blot the coffee, the sooner the better. Also, try this method in a spray bottle, which works well because using less than more is good.

Instead of the gentle remedy for a small coffee stain, I put together a hydrogen peroxide and baking soda mixture. My new off-white rug was bleached white within 20 minutes and ruined for good. But the coffee stain was gone. Opt for the vinegar remedy.

For best results: Be careful and try not to spill coffee. One more thing: Mild laundry detergent mixed with water works well. Use a small amount of soap (a 1 to 4 ratio). Let dry. Forget the peroxide, because it will only lead to bleaching out your item and tears will follow.

HEALTHY COFFEE FENG SHUI TIPS

Welcome your home sweet home to the art of feng shui—the ancient Chinese art of placement—with a twist of coffee. By putting stuff in the right spots in your kitchen and other rooms you can enhance the flow of positive energy and zap negative vibrations, bringing you good health, happiness—and even fortune. Read on—you, too, can enjoy a well-balanced ambiance from head to toe—with a touch of coffee, from room to room.

Declutter Your Coffees. If you're a coffee lover, chances are you're going to have more rather than less java beans and gadgets in your home. Rather than stuffing it all in one place, such as your pantry, I suggest storing it in a variety of places just in case of a blackout. You'll find cans of coffee (these have expiration dates) in my pantry. Plus, they are sealed so I feel safe and secure that my fur kids won't get into the java. Also, when I open my freezer there is an array of well-packaged coffees lined up in rows. It makes me feel safe in case there is a shortage of coffee. And, in my fridge, I also have concealed containers filled with coffee in use, from day to day. It's clutter free, but coffee definitely has its place(s) in my kitchen.

Clean the Coffeepot(s) and Coffee Grinder. This is a chore, but it's good chi to have a squeaky clean pot (or two) and grinder. For the pot, use vinegar, water, and lemon (use hot water, let soak). As far as the grinder goes, day-by-day cleaning will keep you and yours healthy coffee drinkers.

Brighten Up with Lighting. In your kitchen, you'll want to have neutral or earthy coffee colors from a tan, light coffee on wood paneling. Fresh, white curtains will lighten up the room and your energy.

Scent It Up. And, of course, the constant aroma of fresh-brewed coffee will linger from room to room.

Boost Your Mood with Coffee Mugs. Select your favorite coffee mugs and place them together or in a mug holder on the counter. This is inviting for you or coffee.

Use Coffee Art. Framed coffee prints can give your kitchen a nice visual effect, especially if they boast Mediterranean colors: red, brown, gold, and blue.

Flaunt Coffee Companions. Glass canisters filled with from biscotti to coffee candy look inviting and are your friends whenever you decide to brew a cup of java.

Bring Out the Fresh Fruit. Seasonal fruit in lucky numbers, such as eight, is good for you both physically and mentally. Citrus fruit, such as oranges, goes well with coffees—and the shelf life is good.

Conceal Knives and Scissors. These are must-have items so when you open a new bag of coffee you can do it the right way and without going on a hunt through the house or using your nails or teeth.

Hide the Gadgets. Too many coffeemakers will give you clutter. So, choose your coffee toys and store the others in cupboards. Recycle these to fit the season and your mood.

Place Coffee Books in Piles. Cookbooks are attractive and show that you like being in the kitchen. Line these up in an appealing way or pile books in stacks. Either way it will give a nice coffee literary feel and will be on hand to inspire you.

A *Bonus Tip:* Purchase a coffee calendar. It will keep you up-to-date on seasons and holidays—a great coffee lover's tool so you can plan meals and coffee accordingly. And, of course, with your coffeeized kitchen, what better way to celebrate than to have a cake, like this heavenly recipe, baking in the oven?

Heavenly Coffee Angel Food Cake

❖ ❖ ❖

1 cup sifted cake flour
2 tablespoons instant coffee, ground fine powder in a coffee grinder
1¼ cups sugar
½ teaspoon salt substitute

1½ cups egg whites (10–12 large eggs) at room temperature
1 teaspoon of cream of tartar
1 teaspoon vanilla extract
1 teaspoon coffee extract (or almond extract)

Place a rack in the center of the oven and preheat it to 325°F. Sift the flour and ground instant coffee together onto a sheet of wax paper, then resift it with the sugar and salt substitute onto a second sheet of wax paper. In a large grease-free bowl of an electric mixer, add the egg whites and cream of tartar and mix on low speed till foamy. Increase speed gradually to medium and beat until whites are stiff and shiny but not dry. Stop the mixer and add the vanilla and coffee extracts, whisking in once or twice by hand.

Carefully lift the wax paper holding the dry ingredients and sprinkle the flour mixture gently into the egg whites. Using a spatula, carefully fold the dry ingredients into the whites till just incorporated. Do not stir hard or the batter will deflate. Very gently turn the batter into an ungreased tube pan and smooth the top lightly. Place immediately in the oven and bake for 45 minutes or till well risen and golden on top.

As soon as the cake is done baking, invert (if your tube pan doesn't have "feet" hang the pan upside down over the neck of a bottle). Allow the pan to hang upside down for several hours until completely cool. (If it cools right side up, gravity will make it sink and become dense.) To remove pan, slide a long thin knife around the

edge of the pan and the center tube to loosen it. Top
the cake with plate, invert, and lift off the pan.

(*Courtesy:* Coffee Science Source.)

Now that we've put coffee items of all kinds in your home, room by
room, and explained how to use it, take a peek at how coffee, a superfood and household friend, can also be enjoyed to beautify yourself
from head to toe without costing you an arm and leg.

A CUP FULL OF PERKS

✓ Coffee consumption is popular in high school, through college,
middle age, and retirement years.
✓ Countries around the world produce coffee, and harvests differ
in time throughout the year before exporting.
✓ Coffee is a universal beverage and, from coffee bars to coffee production, is a growing phenomenon around the globe.
✓ Usage of coffee in the household, like olive oil, can assist as a
cleaning aid for the kitchen, living room, bedroom, and bathroom
to outdoors as an insect repellent.
✓ Coffee candles are a scent-sational addition to every room in the
house for a comforting and rejuvenating aroma.
✓ Scented candles and coffee feng shui throughout the household
are wonderful and healthful additions that can help balance your
mind, body, and spirit.

The Beauty of Coffee

*Do you know how helpless you feel if you have a
full cup of coffee in your hand and you start to
sneeze?*

—Jean Kerr ("Mary, Mary")[1]

As time passed, I could see myself back in time when I was becoming
well rounded like a seasoned coffee tree on a coffee estate. As a working writer amongst the masses of artists in the San Francisco Bay Area,
I did take time-outs for beauty and play fixes, which included socializing at no-name coffee shops with an artistic flair. They weren't Café
Nervosa or Central Perk (like in the *Friends* and *Frasier* American sit-
coms), but these shops did provide quality time with people that my
mind and body craved. And that time-out can make you feel beautiful
inside and outside.

Shopping with a caffeine fix at Hillsdale Mall on El Camino Real—
The Gap, Macy's, Bed & Bath—was heavenly. Those hot café mocha
lattes in tall 16-ounce glasses with espresso, chocolate syrup, topped
with whipped cream, chocolate shavings, and a straw are coffee to
love. On a Friday night, my best friend and I would meet at a coffee
shop. The mental energy perks followed. Our complaints of the work-
week faded. Thanks to the caffeine buzz, we ended up getting a free
makeup session. Then, it was time to shop. After splurging, we'd go

across the street to Borders Bookstore. We bought a pastry and got another cup of coffee. By 11:00 P.M., it was time to hit the different clubs, whether it was on the San Francisco Bay Peninsula or north to the city. Coffee chat for a night on the town was unforgettable and coffees gave us the nudge to do it all.

THE BEAUTIFYING MYSTIQUE OF COFFEE

I'm hardly alone in discovering the beauty benefits of coffee and its versatile healing powers from head to toe. Since coffee is an antioxidant, it protects the body inside and outside. What's more, its grounds are used to improve the skin, something I have experienced.

Drinking coffee can help you get beautiful on the inside, but treating your body on the outside with its healing powers can make you look and feel great, too. And coffee goes back to different uses by Hawaiians and the Japanese. Both cultures are known to use coffee beauty secrets for reducing wrinkles and improving their skin. In fact, it has been said the Japanese have bathed in coffee grounds fermented with pineapple pulp.

JAVA SPA TREATMENTS

It's no beauty secret that coffee combined with other natural ingredients can enhance your blood circulation, zap stress and anxiety, and help to make your skin feel silky and smoother. Coffee grounds teamed with other natural herbs and extracts can help exfoliate, soften, and even make your skin look firmer and glow. And this is why some spas around the nation and world include coffee in their spa treatments. Here, take a look at some of the popular coffee-based treatments:

Coffee Therapeutic Anticellulite Massage

Coffee extract promotes circulation and tones cellulite-prone skin. Rosemary, mint, and citrus calm the mind and revitalize the spirit while peppermint oil relaxes and refreshes tired muscles. This massage will leave you refreshed and rejuvenated.

Coffee Contouring and Cellulite Wrap

Using the beneficial antioxidant and improved cell metabolism of coffee, the wrap begins with BodyCoffee Polish to exfoliate and refresh the skin to enhance the warm, rich detoxifying body wrap. A hot shower with BodyCoffee Blossom Body Wash is followed by the application of hydrating BodyCoffee Body Lotion.

Coffee Scrub

An exfoliating spa ritual that works wonders on the appearance of cellulite by improving micro-circulation with essential oils and ground coffee while detoxifying the skin with Dead Sea Salts. An intoxicating Body Wash blend will gently rinse away tension; the experience is finished with a soothing application of BodyCoffee Lotion.

(*Courtesy*: Cal-a-Vie Health Spa.)

DIY Recipes from Head to Toe

Do-it-yourself products make it possible and easy to enjoy those pampering health spa benefits in the comfort of your home. And more people—both men and women—are discovering the beauty benefits of coffee, whether they're from the grounds or brewed coffee. Here, take a look at some of the at-home treatments I tried from head to toe and you'll be thanking coffee trees.

Hair

Hair Conditioner for Shine: If you're a brunette, coffee can be your choice of conditioner. A simple-to-do coffee treatment works like this: First, use freshly brewed coffee (not instant), the stronger the better—even espresso. Shampoo and rinse your locks while the coffee cools. Apply the liquid to your wet hair; wait for about 10 minutes. Rinse. Note: Do not try this DIY treatment if you have blond hair or color-treated hair. If you have any hesitation, consult your hairstylist before you do coffee.

Face

Coffee Mask: Since I'm fair and blond, the hair rinse wasn't an option. But I did opt for a java home facial using coffee grounds and an egg white. In a small bowl, I mixed 2 tablespoons of fresh, used coffee grounds from my morning brew. Then, I added one whipped egg white. I applied this on my face and let it set for about three minutes. I rinsed with cold water. Coffee grounds are a super exfoliant, like sugar, and egg white (which I've used before) helps to soften skin.

Skin

Coffee Skin Anticellulite Lotion: Before I showered, I turned to an old favorite—olive oil. I combine extra virgin olive oil with coffee grounds on my upper thighs and buttocks. Being lean, I don't have a lot of cellulite, but most women as they age will get some dimpled fat—and, of course, smoother skin is something that is appealing. After several minutes, I showered. I admit my skin felt softer, but since I don't hunt for cellulite (like I did in my twenties) I cannot honestly say it made a difference.

Coffee Body Wash: The next morning, I went to the shower and tried a coffee exfoliant for my entire body. I combined the morning's coffee grounds with an all-natural body soap. My skin did feel softer than when I use Ivory Soap. But I confess the coffee grounds got me a bit wary considering they might clog the shower drain.

Feet

Coffee Foot Soak: That night, I used coffee grounds with honey. I rubbed the rough and gooey concoction all over my feet. Twenty minutes later, I rinsed my feet in warm water. My heels felt smooth, so I treated myself to a pedicure and painted my toenails with a coffee-colored nail polish.

Both spa treatments and do-it-yourself action can do the job. But it doesn't stop there, especially for bold and beautiful people.

PAMPER YOURSELF

A Day in the Life of a Coffee Lover

If you think coffee spa beauty treatments are just for the rich and famous and DIY homemade coffee concoctions are for folks living on a shoestring, you may be right. There is another option for people somewhere in the middle who want to go coffee for beauty.

One summer day, I was craving a vacation. A surprise UPS package was sitting on my doorstop. The brown box was filled with BodyCoffee products and a cheat sheet card that came with descriptions of each container, including "Awaken your senses in a whole new way" and "Discover what cultures around the world have known for centuries—the skin healing miracle of coffee."

It was the perfect gift getaway. Using prepackaged coffee beauty products (that you can buy online) gives you spa coffee treatments right at home. The following is a luxurious one-day spa plan to relax and rejuvenate your body and mind—like I did.

7:00 A.M. Rise and shine. My day starts with being awakened by raccoons or a stray cat outdoors that woke up my Brittany duo. It was time to get up and take them to the trails for their morning walk. I rinsed my face and washed it quickly with the Energizing Body Bar Revitalize. The product claims include: "The intense, dark-hued blend of ground arabica and peppermint extract does much more than cleanse and tone." Well, still half-asleep I admit I was awake and the aroma of the body bar was nice. Wishing I wasn't a dog lover, just a laid-back cat gal, my sibling and I get a move on with the dogs. Edible coffee is on my mind, but I will wait until I return.

7:30 A.M. Savor a cup of java. Instead of eating a large meal, I enjoy a European type of feast. Now it's time for a new flavored coffee. I brew a pot of Cherry Vanilla Crème (made from Colombian Supremo). In a 12-ounce white coffee cup I pour a cup of hot coffee and splashes of 2 percent low-fat milk. I take the treat back with me (and a homemade bran muffin) and crawl into the warm waterbed. The walked-and-fed dogs follow. I turn on the tube, and log onto the computer to fetch my morning e-mail.

8:30 A.M. Coffee shake it up. Blend a shake (made with organic low-fat milk, premium coffee ice cream, a teaspoon of espresso powder, and ½ teaspoon of vanilla extract). I'm ready to take a long, hot shower.

10:00 A.M. Coffee shower time. First, I light a hazelnut coffee–scented candle. It creates an aromatherapy environment in my cabin-type bathroom. Next, I spray the Revitalizing Herbal Mist. It does what is says it will do: "Coffee extract absorbs odors, while essential oils of rosemary, orange, and mint offer a dose of pure refreshment for the body and environment." I was in heaven believing in the scent of the wonder mist while turning on the shower.

First, I tried the Cleansing Body Wash Enhance. Forget basic soap bars. The words that come with this product convinced me: "Enhance your daily routine with a gentle cleanser for bath or shower. Enriched with antioxidant coffee extract, olive oil and aloe vera, to leave your skin exceptionally soft." Oh my, it was. I was hooked. After, I tried the Invigorating Body Polish. The product claims convinced me to do it: "Indulge in an exfoliating spa ritual that works wonders on cellulite. With dead sea salt, essential oils and ground coffee, it's the ultimate body coffee experience." I may never use my old coffee grounds again.

Once out of the shower and dried off, I couldn't stop. I grabbed the Hydrating Body Balm Soothe. The directions told me it can "soothe dry skin with a Native American recipe thousands of years old—a nourishing infusion of antioxidant coffee extract and hemp seed oil." My body felt rejuvenated and supersoft—ready for the day.

12:30 P.M. Time to get a move on. It's time for the treadmill (usually it's a swim). I eat one chocolate coffee truffle and walk/run for about 20 minutes. This isn't as fun as swimming, but it still provides those feel-good endorphins—and turning on the tunes helps to get into the zone.

1:30 P.M. Eat a healthful lunch. I dish up a fresh egg salad sandwich with tomatoes, and spinach lettuce on whole-grain bread toast. Afterward, I try a store-bought iced coffee. It's not my fantasy, but maybe it takes time to get used to it. Or, making my own may be key.

2:00 P.M. Let the dogs outside. Once back, drink a glass of spring water (or two) and turn to Moisturizing Body Lotion Surround. Living in the mountains at Lake Tahoe reminds me that we don't have a lot of humidity. That means dry skin. So, I tried the lotion on my hands. Again, the product says: "The scent of nature's own aphrodisiac, coffee blossom essence, coffee extract, shea butter and healing herbs leave skin more supple and positively glowing." I use it on my arms and elbows for the effect of it all.

3:00 P.M. Go to work. I prefer going to the laptop for articles, desktop for books. Time spent—three hours. Thinking about the Javabalm SPF 15 Lip Balm, I put it on my lips. Note to self: Do this every day.

6:00 P.M. Eat a coffee-rich dinner. Now that my mind is taxed, it's time to feed my body like spa guests who are provided with awesome spa recipes. Tonight it's the coffee-style chicken. (Check out the entree recipes in chapter 18.)

7:00 P.M. Give myself a foot massage. When I finished dinner, I pampered myself with a foot massage. I tried the Energizing Body Oil Discover and it did what the product words said it would do: "Discover the therapeutic benefits of coffee. Our blend of essential oils (mint, rosemary and citrus) and caffeine soothes aching muscles, improves micro-cellular circulation." (It also helps reduce the appearance of cellulite, or it's supposed to do that. I'll settle for soothing aches and pains.)

9:30 P.M. Coffee break. It's time to watch a film. I cuddle up with Zen cat and Simon and Seth, my beloved Brittanys. I treat myself to a half cup of all-natural premium coffee ice cream.

12:30 A.M. My thoughts are on autumn, when coffee beans are harvested. It's a time when I get ready for the mountain seasonal change (from raking pine needles to ordering wood and stocking the pantry). Coffees—good coffees, all kinds, all flavors—are a welcome addition to my favorite season. It's a time to clean, a time to bake—and coffee can provide the energy to keep on moving.

Whatever season it is or wherever you live, a coffee exfoliating mask will rejuvenate your facial skin and you'll feel good both inside and outside. Try this do-it-yourself recipe and enjoy the aroma of a cup of java.

Coffee Body Scrub

❖ ❖ ❖

2 cup of coarsely ground coffee
2–3 tablespoons massage oil

½ cup raw sugar or sea salt

Mix all ingredients together. Take a hot shower to moisten your skin and open your pores. Using wide, circular motions, rub the coffee exfoliant onto your skin with even pressure. Shower off, pat skin dry, and apply a thin layer of your favorite body lotion.

(Courtesy: Spa Index.)

Now that I've given you my favorite coffee beauty secrets, in chapter 15 ("Specialty Coffee Connoisseurs") it's time to bring out the people behind the coffee bean, from plantation workers and roasters to retailers. These folks behind coffee are connected to nature—a connectedness like trees on a coffee plantation.

A CUP FULL OF PERKS

✓ Coffee treatments at spas, DIY treatments, and ready-made beauty products with coffee can help exfoliate, soften, and help make your skin look and feel softer.

✓ Masks, wraps, manicures, pedicures, and baths infused with coffee are offered at spas in America and around the world.

✓ Coffee boasts antibacterial properties and its ability to hold in moisture can keep your skin from face to feet healthy and smoother.

✓ Java-based treatments include honey with natural plant extracts, essential oils, and other ingredients.

✓ DIY inexpensive coffee beauty treatments are quick and easy to prepare and use.

✓ Store-bought coffee beauty products, which are even more pampering and worth the extra price to get the effects, are available in everything from balms, body oils and polishes, mists, lotions, oils, and more.

1 5

Specialty Coffee Connoisseurs

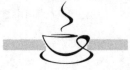

Soup must be eaten boiling hot and coffee drunk piping hot.

—Grimod de La Reynière[1]

Treating myself to a mall coffee and beauty treats was a pampering escape, like a coffee plant getting a nice rain shower. But days like that are not as memorable or as priceless as getting on a jet plane and heading to the Hawaiian Islands—the only state in the United States where coffee is produced—and drinking Kona coffee. And that's what I did when I landed an assignment for a magazine to write about felines on the island of Kauai.

My mission was to interview cat people on the island. I stayed with a cat lady who was a caretaker for more than 80 felines. The morning after my arrival, the sun and the aroma from Mr. Coffee got me out of bed by 5:00 A.M. I wasn't privy to a time-programmed coffeemaker. Sitting in a kitchen with a fascinating hostess who shared stories of the island, cats galore, peacocks outside on the front lawn, and Hawaiian coffee and chocolates to savor by the swimming pool in the backyard were the things that fed my mind, body, and spirit.

THE WORKERS BEHIND YOUR CUP OF COFFEE

While Hawaii is the only state in the United States producing coffee, that doesn't mean other states, including California, don't take part in importing coffee beans and roasting them for coffee lovers. The coffee companies I connected to, whether it was face-to-face or via the phone and Internet in the United States, showed me dedication, passion, and professionalism and their unique coffee made a lasting impression on me and my taste buds.

Alpen Sierra Coffee

Coffee History: As the story goes, in 1988 while on a rainy-day trek near Austria, coffee roaster Christian Waskiewicz was inspired with the vision to create Alpen Sierra Coffee Company in Lake Tahoe. After he had spent much of his life in the Alps of Europe and the Sierra Nevada of California, his dream came to fruition. Serving its first cup of coffee in a historical log cabin on the South Shore of Lake Tahoe in 1991, Alpen Sierra grew to become recognized as the premier roaster of specialty coffees in the Sierra Nevada. Locals and visitors from around the globe can and do enjoy Mountain Roasted Lake Tahoe coffees at home.

In 2007, due to the sluggish economy and high overhead for business owners—and being sandwiched in between one too many Starbucks (think of the film *You've Got Mail,* in which Meg Ryan's character, a small bookstore owner, was forced to shut her doors because of the giant bookstore Fox Books), he had to make a change. Alpen Sierra Coffee Roasting Company relocated to a new and larger roasting facility in the Carson Valley of northern Nevada.[2]

Healing Powers: It's no surprise that the sophisticated roaster embraced the concept and practices of sustainability years ago. In 2002, Alpen Sierra was one of the first specialty micro-roasters in Northern California to become certified organic within the USDA's National Organic Program.

My Fave Coffee: The Hawaiian Hazelnut coffee was one of the best coffees I have tasted during my trek through Coffee World. It could be due to the fact that it was local and superfresh or that the Alpen

Sierra Coffee Roasting Company is an excellent roaster with excellent coffee brokers.

The Colombian Coffee Adventure

Coffee roaster Christian Waskiewicz, founder of Alpen Sierra Coffee, has many exotic coffee tales to share, but one extraordinary trip to Colombia is a standout one. Come along and let him share his traveling adventure, a coffee lover's fantasy, with you. Brew a cup of joe, Colombian preferably, and enjoy:

Invited by Willem Boot to serve as a cupper on a new appellation development project in January '07—this trip promised to be special. Colombia coffees, although showing varied character, mostly through enhanced acidity from select production regions, such as Huila, are familiar and appealing to me for their mild, caramel-sweetness, making them a very accessible and enjoyable cup any time of the day. Arriving in Medellin, the fashion capital of South America, we stayed the first night in a hotel, came together as a group and departed the next day for a mountain-road journey up to Antioquia.

Antioquia is a smallish coffee-producing region located at 2000+ meters SW of Medellin. We were guests of the largest private coffee grower in Colombia, Don Ernesto Garcés, and his daughter, Cristina, who operates their specialty division, Café Montes y Colinas. Our escorts included several federal army and private armed guests, there with us to ensure our safety should any unwelcome trouble arise.

We arrive on a clear and sunny Sunday afternoon in the provincial town of Concordia, where we are welcomed as esteemed guests and treated to a special coffee festival parade, complete with mules with everything from coffee seeding to green coffee bags, precisely balanced to keep the mules moving.

Our team of cuppers consisted of eleven people from several countries: USA, the Netherlands, Panama, Austria, and Colombia. Hotels were not an option in Concordia. In groups of three, we were led to different residences, where we were to be hosted by families of coffee professionals associated with the Garcés family. Meals were prepared by a loving group of ladies and served in one of their humble homes, which was directly adjacent to, and used to be a section of, the town's central church.

With Colombia's production and export being primarily by the FRC, Federal Coffee Control, the program we were here to participate in was to assist the farmers with recognizing and rewarding quality production of "heirloom" varietals, which are then mass-blended prior to export to provide Colombia's well-known "richest coffee" in the world.

The next five days consisted of blind cupping sessions held in a local schoolroom—with a view—experiencing coffees with such extraordinary flavor characteristics as red fruit, passion fruit, high-tone lemony citrus, cacao, Jasmine flower, and coffee blossom.[3]

Coffees of Hawaii

Coffee History: Meet Albert Boyce, owner of Coffees of Hawaii, located on the island of Molokai. He is a fifth-generation member of a family that has worked in partnership with the land since the early 1900s. Its private companies have successfully developed resources including cattle, oil, housing, farming, and ranching in Texas and California over the past century.

Albert enjoys promoting the products of Coffees of Hawaii at sporting events throughout the world, and believes that the beans from this plantation are more than just a commodity. They are part of an island image and lifestyle that is to be healthily enjoyed around the world.

Co-owner Mike Atherton, like Albert (and Christian of Alpen Sierra Coffee), is another man who has a passion for coffee and its roots. Born into a farming, missionary, and political family, Mike entered a world that he fits into, perfectly. He owns and operates a coffee plantation in Nicaragua, Cerro de Jesus (Jesus Mountain). It is located in the Segovia region of northern Nicaragua on the border with Honduras, growing specialty coffee, including several arabica varieties.

The plantation covers about 1,000 acres and has over a million coffee trees.

In September 2004, the Molokai plantation (formerly used for pineapple production) was able to make a complete turnaround with help from Mike and a small group of owners from Manteca, California. They purchased the land on which coffee grew and changed the name of the company from Friendly Isle Coffee to Coffees of Hawaii. The daily breeze and lower precipitation allow this company to grow over-ripened coffee, whereas it's not possible on the Big Island with higher humidity and rain.[4]

Healing Powers: Kona coffee is considered one of the most pricey and extraordinary coffees in the world. Coffees of Hawaii sent me both medium and dark roasts—so while the jury is still out on which beans hold the most antioxidants, I'm covered.

My Fave Coffee: The coffee that intrigued me the most is Kona coffee—known for its pleasing taste and low acidity, it brings me back to the several times I've visited the islands and enjoyed coffee solo and with locals.

It's also their Tisane Coffee Berry Tea that grabbed my attention. Kapalua'u plantation's unique natural dried coffee cherry husks make for a low-caffeine, high-antioxidant creation. Its package description notes: "A ruby-colored cup, deep and mellow in taste, with a softly revitalizing aroma." As a coffee and tea lover, I found Hawaiian Tisane Molokai Style was giving me the best of both worlds.

Meet the Woman Who Has Her Line of Coffee

For Miss Ellie, coffee is the perfect way to pursue several of her passions while assuring that you get the smoothest cup of coffee available. When her stepfather, Bill McClure, wanted her to be part of his gourmet coffee business—Coffee.org—Miss Ellie said, "Sure, but I want to do it the right way, a way where the benefit gets spread around. Oh, and may I have my own line of coffee?"

Miss Ellie has her line of coffee, and the next thing she wanted was direct involvement in choosing the blends that would bear her name. As with all she does, she is demanding and meticulous in the selection process, working closely with her roaster, traveling to out-of-the-way places, testing, tasting, sitting a spell, and reflecting on it.

"In the morning you want a good cup of coffee to get you going and in a good mood to run out the door," she says. "The coffees I choose for Miss Ellie's will definitely do that."

Then there was the business itself. See, Miss Ellie does not believe in ravaging the environment or misusing people. It is probably in the way she was brought up. Raised to do well and do right, she wanted those principles reflected throughout the entire Coffee.org Company. She found the perfect way to do this, through Coffeekids.org, an organization that helps coffee-farming families improve the quality of their lives.

"This isn't about just roasting a bunch of coffee and seeing who wants to buy it," Miss Ellie adds. "I drink my product. I am my own best customer. I hate horrible coffee. I am not going to let anything get to my customers that I don't absolutely love. My name's on the bag, and where I come from, you have pride in your good name."

Ellie Glidewell is a managing partner of Coffee.org. She graduated from the University of Arkansas, Fort Smith, and loved teaching school before deciding to have a coffee named after her.[5]

Coffee.org

Coffee History: Not unlike Coffees of Hawaii, this wholesale coffee products company began with the love of coffee. As the story goes, it is a family-run business. As a retailer for coffee goods, this online company has everything a coffee lover could want, from a wide variety of coffee brands and types to coffee equipment, and so much more. The quality of products is standout and the following is strong.

Healing Powers: When a box of Coffee.org goods was delivered to me, I was greeted with a coffee grinder, a must-have for getting the freshest cup of java. Premium roasts, from organic and fair trade coffee to a bag of flavored dark chocolate mint coffee, were my new coffee friends. Fresh, organic, fair trade—these are some of the things that make coffee drinking a healthful thing to do.

My Fave Coffee: A cup of organic medium-roast coffee was the first organic coffee I have tasted. It's a healthy feeling you get when you eat organic produce. I can't say it tasted different from a non-organic cup of coffee, but the thought behind it is the same reason why I drink organic milk.

Coffee, Tea & Spice

Coffee History: This is another story about a family-run coffee business. Located in Talhina, Oklahoma, in 1994, a gourmet coffee, tea, and spice shop began its online business. They purchase arabica-grade green coffee beans direct from brokers for the best coffee value.[6]

Healing Powers: They roast beans in-house so you are assured the freshest, finest-quality brew. The company also offers shade-grown coffees grown in the understory of the rain forest. They are environmentally friendly, bird friendly, and taste bud friendly. What's more, you can order whole-bean or ground coffee in one-fourth, one-half, and one-pound bags.

My Fave Coffees: Coffee, Tea & Spice offers dozens of flavored coffees. So for me to say one is better than another would be impossible. I have many favorites. Blueberry crumble, Irish crème, cinnamon hazelnut, and Danish pastry come to mind. But that is just off the cuff. Each morning is a pleasure when I turn to one of this company's flavored coffees—it makes the day start off right no matter what news I discover on CNN or my computer. I wish I could give everyone in the world flavored coffees from Coffee, Tea & Spice. It would be a better, more balanced planet.

White Coffee Corporation

Coffee History: When David White contemplated the type of business he would open back in 1939, coffee was mostly consumed for its stimulating effect. When White-Kobrick Coffee Company was formed in 1939, the company specialized in office coffee supply, gradually moving into food service.

Fast-forward to the 1970s, White Coffee decided to dedicate themselves to a category they would help create: specialty coffee. Carole White became president of the White Coffee Corporation in 1992. Jonathan and Gregory White, third-generation family members, continue White Coffee's reputation for the finest-quality products, including a line of flavored coffees.[7]

Healing Powers: White Company, like other coffee companies I've connected with, offers premium coffees, organic, and fair trade.

My Fave Coffees: I preferred flavored varieties and that is what I received. But White Company also carries from White House Exclusives (such as Sury's Personal Blend) to Estate Coffees (like Kenya AA Limited). Pumpkin spice and southern pecan made points with me in the morning, as did the selection of seasonal flavored coffees, including Eggnog, Gingerbread, Hot Buttered Rum, White Coffee Christmas, and Peppermint Crème.

Going Green with Organic Coffee

In order for coffee beans to be labeled as organic they must be grown naturally without fertilizers or pesticides. Furthermore, the processing of the coffee beans must be done without the use of chemicals; this includes the decaffeination process, which typically involves chemicals to remove the caffeine.

Organic coffee can only carry the organic label if it meets the U.S. requirements for being certified, including the land that the coffee is grown being herbicide and pesticide free.

(*Courtesy:* www.coffee.org.)

OUT IN THE COFFEE FIELD

I didn't get to go to Colombia or to Brazil. (My cousin recently moved there if that counts.) I was going to hit the coffee shops around

Lake Tahoe; thought about going back to San Francisco, where coffee-houses made their mark during the Beat era, and overindulging in the beverage menu at Starbucks at our local casino. Then it hit me. Why not pay a visit to one sophisticated coffee roaster who due to the Great Recession and its fallout in our mountain town picked up his equipment and know-how and moved to Minden, Nevada?

By 1:30 P.M., I, and my trusty sidekick-sibling, Bruce, were on the road toward the town of Minden, Nevada, near the center of Carson Valley and just east of Lake Tahoe. I was getting ready to meet the Coffee Man (with 23 years' experience in the coffee industry), who now works about 20 miles away from my home. As Bruce and I were leaving, the lake and towering pine trees were soon replaced by high desert. Then, we were greeted by meadows sprinkled with farmhouses and picturesque cattle.

Not unlike many of our road trips, we took the wrong turn and like two lost homing pigeons made a turnaround. Oddly enough, the environment began to look familiar, much like the peninsula of the San Francisco Bay Area. It was a somewhat sterile high-tech-looking building that caught our eyes as we parked.

Once inside the 4,200-square-foot coffee-roasting building we were greeted by Christopher, a sophisticated coffee roaster and dedicated family man. He took me through the back where roasting machines, coffee bags, boxes, coffee labels, and roasted beans were all around me. Six workers were busy doing what they do, from roasting to turning on the makeshift fan (it was warm).

As we chatted about different roasts and the roasting process (similar to the cocoa beans roasting process, which I wrote about in *The Healing Powers of Chocolate*) I felt a wave of envy. While Christopher **gets his** coffee beans from seasoned brokers around the globe, he did go to Colombia a few years ago. Upon my request, Christopher packaged up some bags of coffee, including Brazil Bobolink and Big Blue Tahoe Blend. These roasts were on my wish list and it made me feel a bit more like a serious coffee drinker. After all, I'd been dabbling in the "girlie" flavored coffees. I was even gifted with two coffee bags with the words "USDA Organic Shade Grown Organic Coffee" from Costa Rica and from Brazil, the latter with a colorful image of a coffee plant with red berries.

Lake Tahoe

One hour later: We were back home by the lake. A quick stop at The Pet Station to pick up fish for my aquariums was on my list. (If I couldn't whisk off to South America, I vowed to give my cabin an exotic effect.)

Once home and settled, I retrieved my e-mail. More flavored coffees and coffee candles are en route to my California home. While images of the classic film *Scarface* came to mind, the scene when character Tony goes to Bolivia, I decide exported coffee and Tahoe will have to suffice. Bruce and I pick up the Brittanys, and by six o'clock we are back home in South Lake Tahoe. . . .

The next morning, I wake up and brew a cup of Brazil Bobolink. (I ground it the night before.) As I sipped the coffee I read the words on Alpen Sierra Coffee Roasting Company's Website: "This semi-washing Brazil offers a deliciously smooth and soft cup. The dark roast degree adds intensity to the medium-bodies, honey-nuanced flavor and spicy finish." This description is spot-on. What's more, I poured another cup. The energizing pick-me-up was amazing.

First, I baked a Cherry Bundt Cake for my *Tahoe Daily Tribune* "What's Cookin' at Callie's Cabin." It was kismet that it used fresh cherries, much like the red coffee berries. I don't often bake in the morning, but I was feeling good. And the physical energy and mental boost lasted throughout the morning. In the afternoon, I treated myself to a slice of fresh cake and a homemade iced coffee to cool down with the warm temperatures.

Coffee Spritzer

❖ ❖ ❖

1 cup Chock full o'Nuts Rich French Roast coffee

1 liter bottle seltzer (without salt) or carbonated mineral water

Pour Chock full o'Nuts Rich French Roast coffee over cracked ice or ice cubes in tall glass with seltzer (without salt) or carbonated mineral water. Serves 1.

(*Courtesy:* Chock full o'Nuts.)

Now that you have met a handful of the hands-on help behind the wide world of coffee trees, it's time to understand that nothing is 100 percent perfect—not even that mug of coffee you drink. There is a downside to java and you should know about it.

A CUP FULL OF PERKS

✓ There are an infinite number of standout coffee companies in the United States and around the world. I connected with companies that promised presentation, originality, and flavor. Not to forget outstanding customer service and knowledge.

✓ Visiting a local coffee roaster or going the extra mile to another town to a coffee company that roasts their coffee is a worthwhile experience both there and when you bring your beans back home. . . .

✓ . . . And finding different coffees from different regions can be done via the Internet with the click of your mouse.

✓ Organic and fair trade coffees encourage a healthier brew and healthier working conditions for the people who are the ones who make it happen to provide you with your coffee choice.

Coffee Is Not Hot for Everyone

Coffee isn't my cup of tea.
—Samuel Goldwyn, American film
producer (1879–1974)[1]

Back in 2006, I was on the road again for work-pleasure. I flew to Southern California for a book tour and stayed at a plush hotel in between Barnes & Noble book lecture/signings. In the morning it was bliss to wake up and ring up room service for a carafe of hot gourmet coffee. But my publicist/gal pal, Kim, ordered decaf coffee because she doesn't like the jolt of caffeine. Decaffeinated coffee, I told her, was a mistake made back in 1903. A German coffee importer, Ludwig Roselius, turned out a batch of Nicaraguan coffee beans that had arrived wet. It was found out by researchers that water had extracted most of the caffeine and left the coffee taste. It was a landmark discovery for decaf lovers.

When our coffee arrived at our hotel room, I sniffed the strong aroma and felt at home while sipping my hot coffee: "How can you wake up to the world without it?" I asked while feeling the elation of a mental and physical boost. But my best friend seemed content with her cup of decaf.

The thing is, there are people who do not like regular coffee for a variety of reasons—and this anticoffee attitude goes back in time and lingers even in the 21st century. Coffee—once tagged as a devil's brew—still has an iffy reputation with some folks as "America's Favorite Drug." Coffee can be a culprit for some people. Here, take a peek at the most common 10 health woes from A to Z and discover what you can do.

Do you freak out at the "caffeine" word? Hate coffee jitters? Can't sleep at night after an afternoon cup of cappuccino? Welcome to the world of fears and anxieties linked to coffee. Don't despair! Brew a cup of regular or decaf and get a grip on what's fact and fiction.

HOW TO BEAT YOUR COFFEE PHOBIAS

1 **FEAR OF HIGH ANXIETY:** Do you ever dread the thought of being anxious to the point of losing control, thanks to the caffeine in coffee? You're not alone, say doctors. It's a big deal if you're prone to anxiety and panic attacks.

   Research has shown that caffeine teamed with emotional stress can raise adrenaline (a hormone that the adrenal glands release in response to stress). Caffeine also blocks adenosine (a brain chemical that has a calming effect) as well as possibly ups muscle tension.[2]

   How to Deal: Coffee is best drunk in moderation (two to three cups per day), so if you're sensitive to caffeine or are on stress overload, curb your caffeinated coffee intake to beat anxiety. The ritual of sipping and savoring a cup of steamy (paired with milk and its calming compounds), flavorful java or an iced coffee can be relaxing. If you're prone to caffeine jitters, switch to half decaf or decaf. Not only will it help you to keep cool, but you'll still get many of the antioxidants and other healing benefits of your coffee fix.

2 **FEAR OF HIGH BLOOD PRESSURE:** While high anxiety or coping with the fight-or-flight response is not fun, placing the BP cuff on your wrist and watching the numbers soar isn't a place you want to be.

   "Caffeine's been shown to increase blood pressure significantly in those who don't habitually use it. The maximum effect occurs fifteen to ninety minutes after consumption, and it can take three to four hours for blood pressure to return to normal," writes *America's Favorite Drug* author. But note, studies show that coffee does not significantly raise blood pressure in people who drink coffee in moderation. In fact, I enjoy one cup of java—all kinds—in the morning. As a human rat experiment I slapped on the BP cuff and my blood pressure numbers read 120/75/55.

How to Deal: If you are prone to high blood pressure, are taking medicines that contain caffeine or phenylpropanolamine, which can raise blood pressure, use common sense. However, if you don't have high blood pressure, or are taking preventative measures to keep it normal, including a heart-healthy diet and exercise, there's no evidence that coffee is going to raise your blood pressure. And in my case it has a calming effect.

3 **FEAR OF HIGH CHOLESTEROL:** On the flip side, do you have a fear of rising cholesterol levels from your favorite cup(s) of coffee? Scientists around the world have found that coffee drinking may be linked to raising cholesterol levels. But the studies vary greatly. For instance, Norwegian studies have found that heavy coffee drinking may raise blood cholesterol up to 14 percent—but some say this increase depends on how the coffee was prepared. One study interviewed 18,000 coffee drinkers; those who made their coffee by boiling it had higher cholesterol levels than those who used other methods—like filtering. And remember, using a French press (no filter) can raise your cholesterol level.

But these Norwegian studies didn't include data about smoking or high-fat diets, which also have a cholesterol connection. Nor did the researchers observe if coffee drinkers turned to black coffee or used cream—another cholesterol link. Interestingly, caffeine doesn't seem to be the culprit, since tea and cola drinkers haven't shown an increase in cholesterol levels, whereas one U.S. study showed that decaf did raise the level of cholesterol. The coffee-cholesterol link could be due to coffee's hundreds of compounds. In other words, the jury is still out to prove that coffee drinking raises bad cholesterol.[3]

How to Deal: To be on the safe side, use a filter method to brew your coffee. It's possible that the filter traps some of whatever it is that hikes cholesterol, or that the coffee grounds don't release as much of it when they're steeped in boiling water. Try eating a heart-healthy diet (whole grain, fruits, vegetables, and low-fat dairy). And yes, drinking coffee in moderation is recommended.

4 FEAR OF DIGESTIVE DISORDERS: If high cholesterol doesn't make your heart race, drinking a cup of acidic java just might. Coffee, much like orange juice, is high in acid, being pH 4.5. Some people are sensitive to acidic beverages and foods and it can cause woes, from heartburn to stomach pain.

How to Deal: Find out about the roasting process of your coffee. Stay clear of darker roasts, which are more likely to cause problems. Also, try half decaf or drink decaffeinated coffee. The water-processed kind doesn't have any added chemicals to increase tummy trouble.

5 FEAR OF EXERCISE: If acidic coffee doesn't bug you, a sobering study may take you back to number 1 anxiety. Researchers from the Utrecht Stroke Center in the Netherlands questioned 250 people about what type of activities they engaged in before having a stroke. Coffee was one of the several culprits on the list, including vigorous exercise that may trigger a hemorrhage stroke caused by a bleed in the brain.

How to Deal: The reality of this fact is that avoiding exercise would be absurd, because this is an activity that keeps our hearts and minds healthy. Drinking one or two cups of coffee and regular exercising isn't stroke material in my book or life. Actually, it provides me motivation to get a move on and my BP numbers are always low after a good swim or dog walk. I'm both energized and relaxed.

Caveat: If you have heart disease and experience irregular heartbeats or other ill effects, stop exercising immediately.

6 FEAR OF FIBROCYSTIC BREASTS: Benign lumps and bumps or cysts in the breasts are a common condition. When I was in my early twenties, my doctor alerted me to the fact that I should be on alert and that more lumps could develop if I didn't stay clear of caffeine. Ironically, as a survivor of PMS I knew coffee in moderation seemed to get me through those days.

How to Deal: America's Favorite Drug author writes in her book: "Switching to decaf won't necessarily help this problem, as decaf contains chemicals like theobromine and theophylline," two bad guys that can aggravate the situation on breasts. It's an individual call, but coffee is energizing, which can lead to exercising and making love—two natural activities that up feel-good endorphins and alleviate pain.[4]

7 **FEAR OF INFERTILITY:** Being able to bear children can be a challenge for both women and men. However, research points to the fact that coffee may lower the odds of conception for women and up the chances for men. Researchers point out that drinking coffee may help increase sperm mobility, but it's a catch-22—because it also may deform sperm, which makes me think of the film sequel to *The Fly*.

Women also are challenged by the fact that caffeine from their bloodstream can penetrate the fertilized egg; right before it embeds in the lining of the womb. In result, this may hinder the blastocyst from implanting—destroying the chances of implanting.

How to Deal: If you're a woman, try switching to half caffeinated coffee or decaf or even eliminating drinking java. (You can still get effects by using it topically for beauty and aroma benefits, as I discuss elsewhere.) For men only: Cut your intake in half, especially if you drink more than three cups of coffee per day. Remember, a little bit of coffee may be a good thing.

8 **FEAR OF INTERSTITIAL CYSTITIS:** As noted in fear number 4, coffee is acidic and the "A" word is poison to women and men who suffer from interstitial cystitis—inflammation of the bladder—a chronic disease of the urinary bladder that creates an urgency to go and pressure on the bladder or pelvis. Coffee is on the avoid list, especially if you have constant flare-ups.

"One of the hardest parts of the IC diet is avoiding these foods that are high in acid, especially coffees and teas. But, if you're addicted to coffee, this can be a shocking blow," says Jill

Osborne, founder of the Interstitial Cystitis Network. She recommends trying a variety of low-acid coffees that are easier on
tender bladders. And you may be able to enjoy a wide variety of
coffees, including Dark French Roast, Hazelnut, House Blend,
and vanilla.[5]

How to Deal: Low-acid coffees are worth a shot. If your cystitis
is mild, try diluting coffee with milk. By trial and error, if you're a
coffee lover, you may figure out if your body can handle coffee.
Keep in mind, moderation is key.

9 FEAR OF INSOMNIA: Cystitis can be a pain, but not getting
adequate shut-eye can be dreadful. We need at least seven hours
of sleep per night to help restore and rejuvenate our bodies and
minds. Coffee with its caffeine can indeed end up being your
best friend if you need to stay up but when you want to sleep it
can get in the way of getting your z-z-z's.

How to Deal: I can personally attest that if I drink one to two
cups of coffee before 3:00 P.M. it provides lots of physical and
mental energy to keep me going throughout the day and night.
Once I hit the sack—I sleep like a baby. However, everyone is different. Some people can enjoy a cup of cappuccino after dinner
and have no sleep disturbances.

10 FEAR OF CUTTING BACK COFFEE: Guru Edwards notes
in her book: "Quitting coffee 'cold turkey'—stopping your coffee
intake all at once—can cause mild to severe headaches as well as
other unpleasant side effects like nausea, anxiety, fatigue and depression. Those are all signs that you've actually been addicted to
coffee."[6]

How to Deal: There are different ways to wean yourself off coffee if you have a reason to do so. One way is to taper slowly, by
cutting back by one cup every few days until you're at the
amount you want to consume, and/or drink half decaf/half regular brew. Also, Edwards recommends including exercise, antistress vitamins (such as B complex and C) and minerals calcium
and magnesium. Plus, since coffee can be a relaxing ritual, try savoring tea (i.e., both black and green tea do contain some caffeine while herbal teas are caffeine free).[7]

THE COFFEE HEALTH DEBATE

Today, despite the groundbreaking studies on the upside of coffee and its perks, there is still controversy on just how much of a health food coffee is. So, I contacted Katherine Tallmadge, R.D., past National Spokesperson of the American Dietetic Association, and she dished out a conservative viewpoint of both pros and cons of java in coffee bean shell.

"Coffee is one of the most confusing foods. It surely contains one of the highest antioxidant contents of all foods, but the research on the health benefits is mixed, so this complicates my recommendation for patients." As a registered dietitian, Tallmadge believes it's her duty to interpret the science and advise her patients how best to eat to improve their health and lives. She quips, "The conflicting research on coffee hasn't made this easy!"

So, the diet expert individualizes her recommendations to her clients, based on their personal needs and medical history. Her advice is much like mine: "Drink in moderation: one to two cups per day" (That's 8-ounce cups!) The bottom line: Tallmadge concludes, "For many people eliminating coffee will make a positive difference in their health. For others, perhaps not. Personalized advice is key to good health."

Kiss Off Coffee Teeth Stains

There is no doubt about it, coffee can and will stain your pearly whites. That includes pricey cosmetic surgery, too, and from bonding to teeth whitening. So, what's a coffee lover to do?

Years ago, I spent hundreds of dollars on bonding for a tooth. During this time I was enjoying coffee—the quality stuff—with my neighbor and friends, too. I didn't want to lose the effect of the bonding, nor stop my coffee breaks. But coffee can stain teeth and it's acidic, like orange juice and vinegar. So, I turned to a couple of tricks that I still put to work these days.

First, I use a straw despite the shape of coffee cup. Next, I'll rinse my mouth with water (if possible) after drinking the dark beverage. And, if at home, sometimes I'll even brush my teeth, especially if the coffee drink is garnished with whipped cream or chocolate. This way, you can have your smile and coffee, too. A bonus tip: Low-acid coffee causes less teeth staining.

ANIMALS AND COFFEE DON'T MIX

Fears of coffee backlash may wreak havoc on your mind and body—but the truth is, dogs, cats, and other animals can also share java jeopardy, too. Like chocolate, coffee in any form contains caffeine and theobromine. If Fido or Fluffy gets into a bag of coffee beans or ground coffee or a fresh cup of brew, trouble may be brewing.

Symptoms of getting into coffee can vary from nervousness, pacing, and vomiting to diarrhea and even seizures. It depends on how much your companion animal consumes and on its weight. Call your veterinarian ASAP if your pet has a coffee moment, because every minute counts. Also, consult with your vet before and find out what you can do if a coffee emergency happens on a weekend or holiday so you can take charge with natural remedies.

So, now that you understand why coffee may not be everyone's cup of tea or if you love it but are hesitant to drink a cup of brew because of its potential consequences, there are ways to have your coffee and eat it, too. This Coffee Cheesecake recipe includes decaf coffee, and a slice of it can be served with decaf, half decaf, or even tea made with the coffee berry.

Coffee Cheesecake

❖ ❖ ❖

1½ cups whole-grain
  graham-cracker crumbs
2 teaspoons almond extract
6 tablespoons butter
  (¾ stick)
1 8-ounce package semi-
  sweet chocolate squares
3 eggs or egg replacement

⅔ cup dehydrated cane juice
  (a type of natural brown
  sugar) or equivalent
  amount of honey
⅓ cup milk or soy milk
2 teaspoons instant coffee
  powder (regular or decaf)
4 8-ounce packages soft
  cream cheese or low-fat
  cream cheese
Almond pieces for garnish

Prepare early in the day. In a 9-by-3-inch pan, use your fingers to mix graham-cracker crumbs, almond extract, and butter; press onto bottom and around the side of the pan. Leave 1 inch from top of the pan to the top of the cracker crumbs. Preheat oven to 350°F. In a small, heavy, stainless-steel iron or titanium saucepan over low heat, melt 6 squares of semi-sweet chocolate, stirring frequently. Add melted chocolate, eggs or egg replacement, cane juice or honey, milk, and coffee; beat until blended. Increase speed to medium; beat 3 minutes, occasionally scraping bowl with rubber spatula. Pour cream cheese mixture into crust in pan. Bake cheesecake 45 minutes; cool in pan on wire rack. Cover and refrigerate cheesecake at least 4 hours or until well chilled. Grate remaining 2 squares of semi-sweet chocolate. Garnish top of cake with grated chocolate and almond pieces. Serves 20.

(*Courtesy:* Lewis Harrison, Director of The Spa of the Mind and B&B; www.theharrisoncenter.com.)

If you have sensitivity to coffee internally, it may work for you topically—for beauty uses or the variety of household uses I provided in a previous chapter. In the future, I sense that coffee—the antioxidant-rich medium and dark roasts—will be used more from kitchens and households to medical clinics and hospitals around the globe. In chapter 17, "The Joy of Cooking with Coffee," you'll be reminded of how important the coffee plant is to our world.

THE HEALING POWERS OF COFFEE

✓ Coffee has been blamed for high anxiety, heart problems, digestive disorders, insomnia, and worse. But there are ways to enjoy coffee without ill effects.

✓ While coffee gets a bad rap for mental and physical woes, it also has been slammed for cosmetic problems—yet there are ways to get around these issues, too.

✓ Pets and coffee do not mix, so coffee lovers must stay on alert and keep their companion animals' paws off any form of coffee products, whether it's fresh brew, beans, candy, or ice cream. Paws off!

The Joy of Cooking
with Coffee

*Chefs often use secret ingredients to add mysterious
depth and nuance to a dish, and coffee is one of them.*
—Corby Kummer, *The Joy of Coffee,* Chapters
Publishing, 1995[1]

I have lived and worked up and down the West Coast—and coffee always played a role in comfort and renewal. In December of 2005, one year after the great Indian Ocean quake-tsunami, a TV crew from India on a *National Geographic* assignment paid me a visit for an interview regarding my book on earthquake prediction and the big wave. I sensed the crew would be tired from their traveling, so I planned to provide an array of eats for a brunch—including coffee.

As a hermitess, I hadn't served four people or made a full pot of fresh-brewed coffee for people in a foreign country, so I was at a loss for the amount of coffee grounds or type of coffee to use. I sensed to use more rather than less would be best. When the crew of four men came into my cabin at noon, I asked, "Coffee or tea?" The word "coffee" echoed loudly from the living room to the kitchen. I was awestruck at how fast the jet-lagged crew drank the java brew—and they were pleased. Later, I discovered coffee is a favorite beverage in India from coffee production to coffee bars. So, my instincts worked. If I had a redo I would have served espresso baked goods.

BAKING WITH ESPRESSO POWDER

Espresso powder is a must-have ingredient if you bake with chocolate. Here's why:

Espresso powder is chocolate's best friend. Use ½ to 2 teaspoons in chocolate baked goods, frostings, and sauces; a touch of espresso powder enhances chocolate's flavor without adding any coffee flavor of its own.

Ground, brewed, then dried from specially selected coffee beans, powder readily dissolves for easy mixing.

For mocha flavor, use 2 teaspoons or more; or use espresso powder on its own to add clean, strong coffee flavor to frostings, bars, cakes, and cookies.

Chocolate and coffee go together like . . . well, like chocolate and vanilla. Both vanilla and coffee highlight chocolate's deep, rich flavor—without imparting any but the faintest hint of their own flavor. Add a teaspoon or two of espresso powder to your favorite brownie, chocolate chip cookie, devil's food cake, or other chocolate recipe, and taste what a difference it makes—your chocolate will sing!

(*Courtesy*: King Arthur Flour.)

THE COFFEE GROUNDS RULES

You, like I did, may think there is nothing to brewing coffee beans and using coffee. Think again. There is a fine art—which is controversial—to tending to keeping coffee. So, I went to the coffee experts to get the scoop, from purchasing to storing. Here, consider these rules from the people who know coffee.

Do purchase coffee as soon after it has been roasted as possible.

Do purchase your coffee fresh every one or two weeks.

Do grind your beans as close to the brew time as possible. (A burr or mill grinder is preferable because all of the coffee is ground to a consistent size. A blade grinder is less preferable because some of the coffee will be ground more finely than the rest.)

Do tell the professionals where you purchase your coffee exactly how you will be brewing it. (For example, will you be using a plunger pot? A flat drip filter? A cone drip filter? A gold mesh filter? They will grind it specifically for the preparation method you have chosen and the equipment you use.)

Do remember to never reuse your coffee grounds. Once coffee is brewed, the desirable coffee flavors have been extracted and only the bitter undesirable ones are left.

Do use filtered or bottled water if your tap water is not good or imparts a strong odor or taste, such as chlorine. Be sure to use colder water.

Do use the proper amount of coffee for every 6 ounces of water that is brewed. A general guideline is 1 to 2 tablespoons of ground coffee for every 6 ounces of water.

(*Courtesy*: National Coffee Association of U.S.A. Inc. Adapted from "How to Brew Coffee.")

MY COFFEE-STYLE SHOPPING LIST

Did you know that coffee—all types, forms, and flavored—can be used for breakfast, appetizers, sauces, entrees, desserts, and non-alcoholic and alcoholic beverages? While coffee isn't included in the Mediterranean Diet Pyramid, you can team it with common Mediterranean foods—as Europeans do. It's a way of life. (In chapter 6, "The Mediterranean Cuppa Comfort," I provide a chart of specific common foods and flavors of the Mediterranean Diet Pyramid. And here I share some of my own spin-off superfoods.)

The first step to Mediterranean cooking is having the right foods on hand. Below you'll find common staples—including coffees—found in Mediterranean kitchens, like mine.

Beverages

Bottled Fruit/Vegetable Juices (100 percent fruit juices): Apple cider is higher in fiber and nutrients than other juices that are more concentrated and processed. You can add a few tablespoons of flavored coffee for a punch.

Coffees: medium- and dark-roast coffee beans (regular and decaf), espresso powder, instant coffee, flavored coffees.

Tea (black, green, herbal): Try flavored tea, such as chamomile, cinnamon, and orange spice. Add to coffee.

Breads and Crackers

Bagels: Go for the small, whole grain, all-natural variety. A bakery bagel can rack up hundreds of calories and preservatives. Perfect with coffee beverages.

Biscotti: Different flavors of all-natural gourmet biscotti. These are ideal with coffees—especially biscotti.

Fig bars, graham crackers (whole wheat): These versatile classics go with coffee as well as crackers and are used in baking.

Whole-grain crackers: Watch for sodium. These can be good for snacks and pair nicely with cheeses, fresh fruit, and coffees.

Canned Foods

Soup: Stay clear of high-sodium soups (e.g., clam chowder). Opt for the low-sodium brands, including chicken rice and vegetable. (During fall/winter, team with a cup of java to get a double dose of immune-boosting antioxidants.)

Marinara sauce: Choose a low-fat tomato-based sauce infused with olive oil. Try to pick an all-natural brand and stay under 400 milligrams of sodium per serving. (Great when teamed with coffee in a sauce with pasta for a kick of flavor.)

Water-packed tuna: albacore tuna in water. (Ideal for a salad with iced coffee in spring/summer; tuna melt and latte in fall/winter.)

Cereals

Oats, whole and quick: Whole is higher in fiber than quick. For a treat, adding a small amount of espresso powder can give this cereal a kick or in baking oatmeal muffins or cookies.

Whole-grain cereal: Look for a vitamin-mineral-enriched brand that has less rather than more sodium. Teaming whole grains with a cup of java in the A.M. will get you plenty of antioxidants.

Dairy

Cheeses: Instead of indulging in large amounts of reduced-calorie cheese, opt for a small amount of real cheese, such as cheddar and mozzarella. Shredded will help you eat less rather than more. Cheese and coffee go together well.

European-style butter: Forget reduced-calorie or diet margarine. Real butter is richer and smoother—better for baking and pairing with coffee—also if used sparingly on breads it's more decadent with a cup of coffee.

Low-fat milk: Opt for low-fat or skim rather than whole milk, which is too high in saturated fat and cholesterol.

Half-and-half: Good for specialty coffee drinks and milkshakes. Use in moderation.

Yogurt: Low-fat or Greek yogurt tastes better than fat-free varieties. Stick to plain and sweeten with honey or coffee. Or try coffee flavored, which has less sugar than fruit yogurts.

Oils, Vinegars, Honeys

Apple cider vinegar: Raw, unfiltered vinegar is best. Good for home cures combined with coffee.

Extra virgin olive oil: The best primary fat to use in your diet regime, including drizzled on food, as a dressing, for cooking and baking. Works for coffee beauty treatments.

Herbs, Spices, Dried Fruits

Fresh herbs: chives, parsley, rosemary, and sage. Ideal in coffee sauces.

Spices: cardamom, cayenne, cinnamon, ginger, nutmeg. Essential for coffee specialty drinks.

Dried fruit: prunes, raisins (black and yellow), cranberries. Good for baking and teaming with espresso powder or instant coffee.

Protein

Eggs: organic, brown. Preferred when baking with coffee.

Frozen Foods

Premium ice cream (coffee varieties often include real coffee and caffeine).

Sorbet (coffee).

MOJO FROM YOUR KITCHEN

Here are some of the best baking and cooking coffee matches at a glance that you should know about before you hit the kitchen. (For more information, go back to chapter 7, "Types of Blends and Roasts.")

Coffee	Flavor	Uses: Baking/Cooking
Colombian coffee		Bagels, breads, cakes, crepes
Costa Rican coffee		Muffins, croissants, butter cookies, eggs
Guatemalan coffee		Cinnamon rolls, coffee cake, cereal, custard
Instant espresso powder	Shot of coffee flavor without extra liquid	Cakes, cookies, chocolaty recipes, enhances cocoa
Dark roasts	Strong	Coffee rub for chicken thighs, dark beef, or lamb
Hazelnut coffee	Smooth, sweet	Coffee cake, chocolate cake
Kona coffee		Coffee cake, cookies, muffins, scones, waffles
Mexican coffee		Muffins, pastries, scones

STORING COFFEE TIPS FOR COFFEE'S SAKE

Scoring quality coffee is a task. Once you have beans (green to roast yourself or roasted ones) that you're proud enough to show off to family and friends (or hide for your eyes only), it's time to store beans the right way. During my time in Coffee World, I learned that there is an ongoing debate about the best way to keep beans fresh. The consensus is keep your beans and grounds airtight. But that's not all. . . .

Keeping your beans fresh in a dark, cool pantry and keeping it in a ceramic container in the fridge or freezer are some of the ways I've been told to do it. It seems to me that storing beans is like storing bread or chocolate. Some people keep it in the cupboard; others put it in the fridge or freezer.

So I've learned that what works for me works. Since I tried and tested dozens of coffees, there was no way in the Coffee World that I could consume a lot all at once, nor did I want to waste quality java. That said, my freezer is stocked with coffees (beans only are best) in airtight bags (a one-way valve to take out the air). Also, there are coffees in cans and coffee pods in boxes in my pantry, too.

You can be the final judge (there is no coffee cop) on exactly how to store your favorite coffee beans to keep them at their best for the freshest cup of brew.

- Freezing is not good for coffee beans.
- The best method to store your fresh roasted coffee beans is with airtight containers. The biggest detriment to keeping coffee beans fresh is exposure to air and moisture.
- It's always best to keep your whole beans fresh and grind just prior to brewing that great cup of coffee.
- Don't order or purchase a huge supply of coffee beans, only to keep them around for an extended period of time.
- Better to buy smaller batches of fresh roasted coffee that you can comfortably consume in about a week's time.

(*Courtesy*: Gourmet-coffee-zone.com.)

Drinking coffee and using coffee in cooking and baking goes way, way back in time. It's a way of life and connecting to people. The *Cooking with the Bible* co-authors point out that while they use foods from biblical times, they also made use of many foods that have more recently become common in Middle Eastern fare: "More important than the exact reproduction of a dish or a meal is the spirit in which it is prepared and served. In biblical times, an invitation to dine, whether with family and friends or with complete strangers, was taken seriously." Here, this tantalizing recipe will entice you to enjoy the adventure of cooking and baking on the long coffee bean road.

Salome's Honey-Carob Brownies

❖ ❖ ❖

¾ cup flour	⅓ cup carob powder
1 teaspoon baking powder	1 cup bee honey
¼ teaspoon salt	2 eggs
¼ teaspoon mace	½ cup fresh-brewed coffee
¼ cup oatmeal	½ cup pistachios, chopped
⅔ cup butter	1 teaspoon almond extract

Preheat oven to 300°F. Sift together the flour, baking powder, salt, and mace. Stir in the oatmeal. Melt the butter in a small pan over low heat. Add carob powder and honey and blend well, removing from heat in a mixing bowl, then beat the eggs and gradually add the carob mixture. Add the coffee, pistachios, and almond extract and mix well. Pour into an oiled 8-inch-square pan and bake for about 35 minutes or until done Yield: 2 dozen brownies.

(Courtesy: Cooking with the Bible: Biblical Food, Feasts, and Lore by Anthony F. Chiffolo and Rayner W. Hesse, Jr. Copyright © 2006; reproduced with permission of ABC-CLIO, Santa Barbara, CA.)

Now that you've learned everything you want to know about healing coffee (from history, types, and health benefits to home cures and beauty and household hints) but were afraid to ask, it's time to bring in the recipes made with coffee or ideal to pair with a coffee beverage for your new, improved life, in part 8, "Coffee Recipes."

A Cup Full of Perks

✓ Learn the tips to baking with espresso powder before you bake up a dish.

✓ There are tips to brewing coffee so you'll enjoy the most flavorful, fresh cup of java.

✓ The coffee storage debate is ongoing, but there are basic facts that coffee lovers abide by to give them the best cup from their beans.

✓ A Mediterranean foods grocery list paired with coffees is something coffee lovers may find essential.

✓ There is an art to pairing the best coffees with foods for cooking and baking so your dishes will be the best that they can be.

PART 8

COFFEE RECIPES

Here Comes the Coffee

*Only Irish coffee provides in a single glass all four
essential food groups: alcohol, caffeine, sugar and
fat.*

—Alex Levin[1]

Unlike the afternoon with a TV crew from India full of hustle bustle
and limelight jitters, I recall another coffee experience. It was off-
season at Lake Tahoe. After an early hot cup of black Italian Roast and
a quick shower, I was off to swim at my favorite resort outdoor swimming pool—despite the snow flurries and brewing snowstorm. Sure,
the sky was gray, but the water was warm with steam rising into the 13-
degree air. Once I got into the zone only my head was cold. I was energized. The staff begged me to come back inside, but I prolonged my
solo swim. Once I got out I scurried on the cold, icy cement up the
stairs to the hot tub. Ah, it was utopia, like the cup of joe that began
my day.

Once I had my thrill swimming in the snow, I got dressed and hit
Starbucks. I ordered a Pumpkin Spice Latte with espresso, pumpkin,
spices, steamed milk, and no whipped cream. Then, it was straight
into the casino room and straight for the Wheel of Fortune slot machines. Twenty dollars later, I heard the "ding, ding, ding" song of the

machine and it paid out $300. With coffee in hand, and cashing out, I was physically and mentally content.

Back home I took the Brittany duo outdoors for a walk as the storm was coming in. After, I brought in several pieces of wood and started a fire. Then, it was to the kitchen. Feeling energized from the swim, coffee, gambling spree, dog walk, and warm fire, I was ready to bake.

You, like me, have entered your kitchen—a place where you can now savor coffee for breakfast, appetizers, main entrees, and desserts. While I sprinkled tried-and-true recipes throughout *The Healing Powers of Coffee*, I saved more than 50 eye-opening coffee dishes (including breakfast, appetizers and breads, entrees and desserts), from seasoned chefs at spas, the National Coffee Association of U.S.A., Inc., brand-name coffee companies, and a few of my own favorite tried and tested creations. For best results, use the coffee type noted in each recipe. Here is a sample of how I incorporate coffee into my daily regime year-round.

THE FOUR SEASONS COFFEE LOVERS MENU PLAN

This four-day coffee diet plan is based on the seasons and a nutritious and natural diet plan to use. Yes, like a coffee tree, you can be nourished and productive too! Recipes can be found at the ends of previous chapters or in this chapter. You can mix and match to suit your personal taste. The recipes with an asterisk can be found in this chapter, or at the ends of other chapters in this book (and feel free to pull a switcheroo to fit your mood and coffee).

Winter: Day 1

Breakfast:
1 Hazelnuts Espresso Biscotti*
2 scrambled eggs with cheddar cheese
1/2 cup cranberries, fresh (drizzled with honey)
1 cup of fresh-brewed coffee

Lunch:
2 ounces feta cheese and $1/2$ cup leafy spinach topped on a whole-
wheat pita pocket with $1/2$ sliced tomato, microwaved till crispy
and hot
1 cup Greek plain yogurt with slices of fresh seasonal fruit

Snack:
Dark chocolate–covered espresso beans
Fruit

Dinner:
Thai Coffee Spiced Chicken Sates*
$1/2$ cup green peas
1 sweet potato

Snack:
A cup of hot chocolate with coffee

Spring: Day 2

Breakfast:
Coffee Cream Blueberry Scones*
Café mocha with skim milk
1 banana

Lunch:
Tuna fish sandwich with tomato slices
1 cup homemade vegetable soup
1 cup fresh fruit salad
1 espresso

Snack:
1 slice Orange Olive Bread*
1 cup herbal tea

Dinner:
Coffee Pork Chops*
Tossed green salad with vinegar and olive oil dressing
French bread and olive oil

Snack:
Fresh fruit over coffee ice cream

Summer: Day 3

Breakfast:
Cappuccino Biscotti*
1 bowl of cold cereal and fresh fruit
1 cup coffee or herbal tea with 1 teaspoon honey
1 glass fresh orange juice

Lunch:
1/2 cup rice
1 cup Greek honey yogurt
Iced cappuccino

Snack:
Fresh fruit

Dinner:
Prawn Mole*
Mixed vegetables
1 whole-grain roll

Snack:
Chocolate coffee truffles or chocolate coffee bar*
1 espresso (decaf or regular)

Fall: Day 4

Breakfast:
Pumpkin Spiced Coffee Muffins*
1 cup skim or low-fat milk
6 ounces fresh orange juice
1 cup café mocha

Lunch:

   1 slice organic vegetarian pizza with whole-wheat crust
   1 cup leafy spinach salad with tomatoes, carrots, red wine vinegar
      and olive oil dressing
   1 cup coffee Greek yogurt with sliced apples

Snack:

   1 cup of cruciferous vegetables, raw
   1 Pumpkin Spice Latte

Dinner:

   Coffee Chili*
   Cornbread spread with honey
   ½ cup green vegetable

Snack:

   1 slice Heavenly Coffee Angel Food Cake*
   1 cup decaf flavored coffee

A Coffee Buzz on How Much to Eat: Like Europeans, I do not count calories. However, I do rely on portion control—I eat small meals on small plates—to keep my calories in check. (And I do not eat after 7:00 P.M.) Read food labels and you'll see how easy it is to decode one serving size and its ingredients (i.e., cholesterol, fat, sodium, etcetera) and if it's natural or includes artificial stuff. But note, serving sizes also depend on activity level, size, gender, and age. Don't forget, most health organizations recommend at least 5 servings of fruits and vegetables per day. If the recipe doesn't include serving sizes, use your own judgment and stay on portion control watch.

Breakfast

On a dark, stormy midnight in the California sierra, I walked outdoors into the cold with my two Brittanys. The front deck was covered with wet snow; the towering trees and wires amid me looked surreal and eerie because they were wilted with white powder. I shoveled the heavy slush off the deck to make it easier for the morning. At 7:30 A.M. I got out of bed and turned on the TV switch for CNN—there were no red and amber lights on the cable box. I flicked on the lamp—it didn't work. "Power outage," I mumbled. It was the beginning of the first day the lights went out at South Lake Tahoe.

Instead of making a cup of fresh-brewed java with my electric coffee-maker, I turned on the gas burner and grabbed a jar of instant coffee. (I said a prayer to chemist Satori Kato for his invention.) The first taste of the stuff I used to drink was doable but nothing to write home about and did its job. Once alert I got my first news report from a neighbor walking her dog. "The power will be out for days," she shouted. Her words echoed in my mind. I tuned out her warning. I hoped for the best, but by dusk I went into survival mode and prepared for the worst. Read: more instant coffee. Making and storing gourmet coffee and from coffee croissants to coffee cakes, like these, will make your days sweeter no matter what challenges you face.

Apple Almond Croissants with Coffee Glaze
Cappuccino Biscotti
Cinnamon-Cappuccino-Pecan Scones
Cinnamon Coffee Rolls
Coffee Cake
Coffee Cream Blueberry Scones
Kahlúa Biscotti
Pumpkin Spiced Coffee Muffins
Yogurt Coffee Cake

Apple Almond Coffee Croissants with Coffee Glaze

❖ ❖ ❖

1 tube refrigerated large croissant rolls
4 Fuji apples, peeled and chopped
3 tablespoons European-style butter

½ teaspoon cinnamon
4 tablespoons 2 percent low-fat organic milk
½ cup almonds, sliced

GLAZE

¼ cup orange honey

¼ cup European-style butter, soft

1 teaspoon instant coffee powder

Confectioners' sugar

Pop open package of store-bought rolls. On a flat surface unroll the precut eight triangle-shaped dough pieces. Meanwhile, on medium heat in a saucepan, sauté apples in butter till tender. Add sugar and spice. Put two dough pieces together (to make four croissants) and spread with apples. Roll into croissant shape. Brush with milk. Place each one on an ungreased pan; bake at 350°F for about 15 to 20 minutes or till golden brown. While baked croissants are still in oven, in a saucepan melt honey, butter, and coffee to drizzle on them. Sprinkle generously with almonds. Cool. If preferred, dust with confectioners' sugar. Serves 4.

Cappuccino Biscotti

❖ ❖ ❖

These low-fat cookies are enhanced by the strong coffee that gives them great flavor. Enjoy one of these crispy confections with a cup o'joe or a low-fat latte for a guilt-free afternoon treat.

2 cups flour

1 cup sugar

½ teaspoon baking soda

½ teaspoon baking powder

½ teaspoon salt

½ teaspoon cinnamon

5 tablespoons brewed espresso, cooled

4 teaspoons milk

1 large egg yolk

1 teaspoon vanilla

¾ cup pecans chopped, coarse

½ cup semi-sweet chocolate chip

Stir together in a large bowl the flour, sugar, baking soda, baking powder, salt, and cinnamon till mixed well. In a small bowl, whisk together the espresso, milk, egg yolk, and vanilla. Add liquid mixture to flour mixture and beat till dough forms. Stir in nuts and chips.

Knead the dough on a floured surface till no longer sticky, then halve the dough. Flour your hands and shape each piece into a flattened log 12 inches by 2 inches and arrange the logs at least 3 inches apart on a greased cookie sheet. Bake at 350°F for 35 minutes. Let cool 10 minutes, then cut biscotti on the diagonal into 3/4-inch slices. Arrange biscotti cut side down on the sheets and bake 5 to 6 minutes on each side till they are pale golden. Makes about 40 biscotti.

(*Courtesy:* Coffee Science Source.)

Cinnamon-Cappuccino-Pecan Scones

❖ ❖ ❖

3 cups King Arthur Mellow Pastry
   Blend or Unbleached All-
   Purpose Flour
2 teaspoons baking powder
½ teaspoon baking soda
¾ teaspoon salt
1 teaspoon ground cinnamon
¼ cup granulated sugar
½ cup butter, cut into pats or
   small cubes
⅓ cup pecans, processed or
   blended till very finely ground

½ cup cinnamon chips or
   cinnamon Flav-R-Bites
½ cup cappuccino chips
2 teaspoons espresso powder dissolved in 1 tablespoon hot water[8]
½ cup sour cream or yogurt
   (low-fat is fine)
4 to 5 tablespoons ice water
2 tablespoons coarse white
   sparkling sugar, for topping

Preheat the oven to 400°F. Lightly grease (or line with parchment) a large baking sheet. Whisk together the flour, baking powder, baking soda, salt, cinnamon, and sugar. Work the butter into the dry ingredients till the mixture is unevenly crumbly; don't be afraid to leave some of the butter in pea- or marble-sized chunks. Add the ground pecans and chips, stirring to combine. Dissolve the espresso powder in the hot water. Gently stir the dissolved espresso and sour cream or yogurt into the dough, just till it's well dispersed; the dough will be very crumbly. Add enough ice water to bring the dough together in a cohesive mass.

Gather the dough into a ball, and place it on a well-floured work surface. Pat/roll it into an 8- to 9-inch circle about ¾ inch thick. If desired, brush the surface of the dough with milk, and sprinkle with coarse white sparkling sugar. Use a 2-inch cutter to cut about 20 scones, gathering the scraps and gently shaping into round scones without re-rolling. Place the scones on the prepared baking sheet, leaving just over 1 inch between each. Bake the scones for about 20 minutes, till they're golden brown. When you break one of the center scones open, the middle should be baked all the way through, not doughy or wet. Remove the scones from the oven, and serve warm. Yield: 20 small scones.

(*Courtesy:* King Arthur Flour.)

Cinnamon Coffee Rolls

❖ ❖ ❖

*1 package of large-sized wheat
  crescent rolls*
¼ cup European-style butter
¼ cup light brown sugar

3 to 4 tablespoons cinnamon
½ cup walnuts, chopped
¾ cup raisins

Preheat oven to 350°F. Pop open crescent rolls, unroll dough, and separate into rectangles. Place dough on a cookie sheet or flat dish. Seal serrated edges and brush melted butter on top. Sprinkle sugar and cinnamon mixture. Top with nuts and raisins. Roll up beginning with short end. Cut into slices. Place each circle down and snug as a bug in an 8-by-8-inch baking dish. Bake for 25 minutes or till golden brown. Cool. Drizzle with coffee frosting. Makes 12 petite rolls.

COFFEE FROSTING
¼ cup European-style butter
*1 cup confectioners' sugar (add
  more sugar for desired consistency)*

*½–2 teaspoons strong brewed,
  cooled coffee*
½ teaspoon pure vanilla extract

Melt butter on low heat and add sugar, coffee, and vanilla. Frost tops of rolls.

Coffee Cake

❖ ❖ ❖

1 cup unsalted butter, cut into
   1-inch pieces
1 cup unsweetened cocoa powder
   (plus 2–4 tablespoons for dusting)
1½ cups brewed Chock full o'Nuts
   coffee
½ cup rum

2 cups sugar
2 cups all-purpose flour
1¼ teaspoons baking soda
½ teaspoon salt
2 large eggs
1 teaspoon vanilla

Preheat oven to 324°F. Butter 10-inch cake pan well, then dust with 2–4 tablespoons cocoa powder, knocking out the excess.

Heat coffee, rum, butter, and remaining cup cocoa powder in a 3-quart heavy saucepan over moderate heat, whisking, until butter is melted. Remove from heat, then add sugar and whisk until dissolved. Transfer mixture to a large bowl and cool.

While chocolate mixture cools whisk together flour, baking soda, and salt. Whisk together eggs and vanilla separately, then add to the cooled chocolate mixture until combined well. Add flour mixture and whisk until combined. Pour batter into cake pan and bake until a wooden pick or skewer inserted in center comes out clean, 40 to 50 minutes. Cool cake completely in pan on a rack, about 2 hours.

(*Courtesy:* Chock full o'Nuts; www.chockfullonuts.com.)

Coffee Cream Blueberry Scones

❖ ❖ ❖

2¾–3 cups 100 percent natural
   whole-wheat flour
¼ cup brown sugar
1 teaspoon baking powder
1 teaspoon baking soda
1 teaspoon allspice
¼ cup European-style butter
   (cold cubes)
½ cup sour cream

1 brown egg
¾ cup 2 percent low-fat organic
   milk
2 tablespoons flavored brewed coffee
2 tablespoons flavored honey
1 teaspoon vanilla extract
1 tablespoon orange rind
1½ cups fresh blueberries

Preheat oven to 375°F. In a bowl, mix flour, sugar, baking powder, baking soda, spice, and flavoring. Add chunks of butter, sliced in small cubes. In another bowl, combine sour cream, egg, milk, coffee, honey, vanilla and stir till a dough-like mixture forms. Fold in rind and berries. Drop spoonfuls onto a parchment-lined cookie sheet. (Or, you can also form into a ball, roll out, and cut into ½-inch triangles or circles to achieve that bakery-perfect look.) Bake till brown, about 15 minutes. Makes 12 medium scones. Slice and serve warm with cream cheese or honey and coffee.

Kahlúa Biscotti

❖ ❖ ❖

⅓ cup cocoa
2 teaspoons baking powder
1½ cups sugar
3 cups flour
1 teaspoon salt
1 teaspoon instant coffee powder
Grated peel of 1 orange

3 eggs or 1 egg and 4 egg whites
⅓ cup Marsala Olive Fruit Oil
1 teaspoon vanilla
6 tablespoons Kahlúa liqueur
½ teaspoon almond extract
¾ cup milk (or dark) chocolate chips
1 cup almonds, sliced or ground

In mixing bowl add dry ingredients; make a well in center. In another bowl add eggs, oil, vanilla, Kahlúa, and almond extract; stir. Pour egg mixture into flour mixture, stir until dough holds together, add nuts and chocolate chips. Place dough on floured board; cut into 4 to 6 pieces. Roll each piece into a log 1½ to 2 inches by 10 to 12 inches long. Place on foil-lined greased cookie sheets, 4 inches apart. Bake in 350-degree oven for 20 minutes or until firm to the touch. Remove from oven; let cool about 15 minutes. Using a serrated knife, cut each log diagonally into ½- to- ¾-inch-wide slices. Place biscotti back on cookie sheets cut side down, for 8 to 10 minutes. Makes about 60.

FROSTING

Melt ¾ cup milk (or dark) chocolate chips. Spread a thin layer on one cut side of biscotti. Place on wire rack to firm.

(*Courtesy:* Gemma Sanita Sciabica, *Baking with California Olive Oil: Dolci and Biscotti Recipes.*)

Pumpkin Spiced Coffee Muffins

❖ ❖ ❖

1¾–2 cups all natural whole-
    wheat flour
1 teaspoon allspice
1½ teaspoons baking powder
½ cup brown sugar
½ teaspoon baking soda
1 teaspoon espresso powder
2 teaspoons pumpkin pie spice

1 cup canned pumpkin pie filling
¼ cup sour cream
¼ cup pumpkin spice coffee,
    brewed
2 eggs, brown
1 tablespoon clover honey
1 teaspoon pure vanilla extract
Organic brown sugar

In a bowl, combine dry ingredients. In another bowl, mix pumpkin, sour cream, coffee, and beaten eggs. Add honey and vanilla. Use an ice-cream scoop and place one scoop each into cupcake tins lined with cupcake papers. Bake at 350°F for about 25 minutes or until golden brown and firm. Sprinkle with organic raw sugar.

FROSTING

For a fall and/or Halloween treat: Mix ¼ cup melted cappuccino chips, 1½ cups confectioners' sugar, ¼ cup half-and-half low-fat organic milk, and ½ teaspoon pure vanilla extract. Frost cooled muffins.

Yogurt Coffee Cake

❖ ❖ ❖

1 cup plain yogurt
1 teaspoon baking soda
¼ cup butter or margarine, soft
1 cup lightly packed brown sugar
1 egg

1 teaspoon instant coffee, dissolved
    in 3 tablespoons hot water
1½ cups all-purpose flour
2 teaspoons baking powder

INGREDIENTS FOR MIDDLE LAYER AND TOPPING

½ cup lightly packed brown sugar   1 tablespoon cinnamon
1 tablespoon cocoa

Mix yogurt and baking soda together in a bowl. It will increase in volume immediately. In a separate mixing bowl, cream butter with brown sugar until creamy and light. Beat in egg well; add hot instant coffee mixture. Mix well. Stir the flour and the baking powder together. Alternately add flour and yogurt mixtures to the creamed butter/sugar. Mix carefully but thoroughly.

MIDDLE LAYER AND TOPPING

Pour (spread) half the cake batter into an 8- or 9-inch cake pan (greased). Sprinkle half the topping mixture over top. Bake at 350°F for about 35 minutes or until skewer comes out clean. Cool and serve.

(*Courtesy:* The Roast and Post Coffee Company.)

Appetizers and Side Dishes

While a power outage and sipping generic instant coffee can feel like the end of the world, it was nothing in comparison to what followed. On March 11, a 7.2 hit offshore Japan; followed by a 9.0 and a tsunami that rocked the world. Yes, I did predict 8.0 plus tsunamis would hit in the Pacific Ring of Fire in 2011. At 4:00 A.M. I received a call from *The Mancow Show*'s producer. I was up all night following the catastrophe and manning my earthquake prediction Website— coffee helped. But when the phone rang my awareness level was lukewarm like a cup of stale coffee when the producer noted my Japan quake forecast had come true. I mumbled, "I know." I said I'd call back. After I hung up, I turned on Mr. Coffee. It was this and a beignet that got me through the interview.

The secret to getting energized fast is to turn to coffee and a healthful appetizer—not a big meal. For instance, sipping a cup of hazelnut medium roast with a beignet or enjoying a savory tuna croissant with a cup of espresso will perk you up—and you'll be ready to tackle work or play no matter what's on your day's agenda.

Beignets
Coffee-Infused Dirty Rice
Hazelnuts Espresso Biscotti
Orange Olive Bread
Tuna Italian Croissants
Orange Sweet Potatoes

Beignets

❖ ❖ ❖

¾ cup water
1 tablespoon sugar
½ cup evaporated milk (low fat)
1 package dry yeast (¼ ounce)
3 to 3½ cups flour
1 teaspoon salt

Confectioners' sugar
⅓ cup sugar
½ teaspoon cinnamon, cardamom,
  or nutmeg
2 egg whites
2 tablespoons Marsala Olive Oil

In a small saucepan, over low heat, combine water, 1 tablespoon sugar, and milk; heat to 110°F. Stir in yeast; let stand about 10 minutes. In large mixing bowl, combine dry ingredients. Make well in center; add yeast mixture, egg whites, and olive oil. Stir until dough holds together. Turn dough onto lightly floured surface; knead until smooth. Place back in lightly oiled mixing bowl, cover, and let rise to warm place until doubled in bulk. Turn dough out on lightly floured surface; pat or roll dough out into a rectangle about ½ inch thick. Cut dough into 2-inch-wide strips. Cut strips into 2-inch-wide diamond shapes. Place diamonds 1 inch apart on lightly oiled baking sheets. Cover loosely and let rest about 20 minutes. In saucepan, heat 2 inches olive oil. Carefully slide beignets into hot oil 3 or 4 at a time; do not crowd. Cook until deep golden on both sides. Remove with slotted spoon. Sprinkle with confectioners' sugar. Notes: Dough may be made in food processor. Makes 36.

(Courtesy: Cooking with California Olive Oil: Popular Recipes, Gemma Sanita Sciabica.)

Coffee-Infused Dirty Rice

❖ ❖ ❖

¾ cup brewed coffee
1 cup chicken broth
1 teaspoon dried oregano

1 tablespoon unsalted butter
¼ teaspoon kosher salt
1 cup long-grain rice

In a medium pot, combine the coffee, chicken broth, oregano, butter, and salt. Bring these ingredients to a boil, and add rice while stirring well. Reduce heat to low, and cover the pot and cook until the rice is soft: 18 to 20 minutes. Remove the dish from heat, and serve while it is warm.

(*Courtesy:* ChugginMcCoffee, The Coffee Bump.)

Hazelnuts Espresso Biscotti

❖ ❖ ❖

Biscotti is enjoyed for breakfast, an afternoon snack, and dessert— all with coffee. To me, this nutty biscotti is a perfect appetizer throughout the day.

1 cup hazelnuts chopped coarsely
2 eggs (or 4 egg whites)
5 tablespoons Marsala Olive Fruit Oil
4 teaspoons hazelnut liqueur
2½ cups flour
1½ teaspoons baking powder

1 teaspoon salt
1⅓ cups brown sugar packed
2 tablespoons espresso coffee powder
Grated peel of 1 orange
2 tablespoons orange juice (if needed)

Line baking sheets with foil; grease lightly. On baking sheet toast hazelnuts 5 to 8 minutes in a 325-degree oven; cool. In small bowl stir together eggs, olive oil, and liqueur. In larger mixing bowl combine dry ingredients. Make well in center; pour in egg mixture. Stir with large spoon until dough holds together. Add nuts and peel. Place dough on floured board; cut 3 or 4 inches apart. Bake in a 350-degree oven for about 20 minutes or until firm to the touch. Remove from oven; cool about 15 minutes. With serrated knife cut each log diagonally into ½-inch-wide slices. Place biscotti back on baking sheets, cut side down. Bake 8 to 10 minutes to crisp; cool. Spread one cut side of biscotti with frosting. (Optional: A cup of coffee is recommended.) Makes 50 to 60.

(*Courtesy:* Gemma Sanita Sciabica, *Baking with California Olive Oil: Dolci and Biscotti Recipes.*)

Orange Olive Bread

❖ ❖ ❖

A few years ago, I paid a visit to Frantoio Ristorante near Mill Valley, California. It was the first time I tasted olive bread and the first time I dipped bread into olive oil. The experience was a bittersweet one. I took the bread back to my hotel room. In the morning, when I had a cup of Italian Roast coffee I nibbled on the olive bread and it grew on me. It was a perfect pair.

1 package dry yeast
1 cup orange juice
3 cups flour
1 tablespoon salt (or to taste)
Black pepper to taste
1 tablespoon sugar or honey

6 black olives, chopped
1 tablespoon fresh rosemary, finely
  chopped
¼ cup Sciabica's or Marsala Extra
  Virgin Olive Oil

FOR THE TOPPING
10 whole black olives
1½ tablespoons fresh
  rosemary

2 tablespoons Sciabica's or Marsala
  Extra Virgin Olive Oil
½ teaspoon sea salt (or to taste)

In small mixing bowl, combine yeast with orange juice. In large mixing bowl, add dry ingredients; make well in center. Pour in yeast mixture and olive oil. Stir to blend well, cover, let stay in warm place until doubled. Turn out on lightly floured surface, put down, and spread chopped olives over dough. Knead in olives; make dough into a round loaf. Place in a lightly greased 2-quart baking pan. Lightly press in whole olives and rosemary; drizzle top with olive oil. Let rise until doubled in bulk. Bake covered with foil in a 400-degree oven for about 30 minutes. Uncover; bake 15 to 25 minutes or until golden brown.

Appetizer: Slice bread into ¼-inch slices. Drizzle with olive oil; add one or two anchovy fillets, chopped tomato, and a sprinkle of balsamic vinegar. Add fresh basil leaves and sliced Telene cheese, if desired. These are best prepared as eaten, rather than ahead of time. Makes about 1- to 1½-pound loaf.

(*Courtesy:* Gemma Sanita Sciabica, *Cooking with California Olive Oil: Recipes from the Heart for the Heart.*)

Orange Sweet Potatoes

❖ ❖ ❖

3 medium sweet potatoes, peeled
4 medium oranges
1/4 cup extra-strength coffee
2 tablespoons unsalted butter
1/2 cup chopped, blanched almonds
2 tablespoons dark rum
1 teaspoon baking powder

1/4 cup brown sugar
1/4 teaspoon ground cinnamon
2 tablespoons grated orange zest
Salt and pepper to taste
Fresh mint sprigs for garnish
Slivered, blanched almonds for
  garnish

Cut sweet potatoes into 1/2-inch pieces and drop into a pot of boiling salted water. Cook until just tender, about 15 minutes. Meanwhile, cut the oranges in half and scoop out the fruit. Discard the pulp and juice (or save for other uses). Set the orange shells aside. Remove the cooked potatoes from the heat, drain, and put through a ricer or place in the bowl and mash with a potato masher. Place the mashed potatoes in a warmed bowl. Add the coffee, butter, almonds, rum, baking powder, sugar, cinnamon, and orange zest to the potatoes and mix thoroughly. Salt and pepper to taste. To serve, mound the sweet potato mixture in the 8 orange shells. Garnish each filled shell with a sprig of mint and blanched almonds. Serve at once. Serves 8.

(*Courtesy:* The Roast and Post Coffee Company.)

Tuna Italian Croissants

❖ ❖ ❖

16-ounce can albacore tuna
  packed in water
1/8 cup French Roast coffee, brewed
1/4 cup celery, chopped
1/4 cup green or red bell pepper,
  chopped

2 teaspoons red onion, chopped
2 cups spinach lettuce leaves
2 tablespoons mayonnaise
2 teaspoons red wine vinegar
1/2 cup cheese (feta or mozzarella)
1 package store-bought croissants

Combine tuna with coffee. Add vegetables, mayonnaise, vinegar, and cheese. Place on croissant squares, roll into a crescent shape, and bake according to package directions till golden brown. Serves 4.

Entrees

As a Californian, I have endured from earthquakes to snowstorms—and entrees in between have often been light meals, since I'm a grazer. During the 1989 World Series earthquake, sleep deprivation hit because of the aftershocks and deadlines as a journalist writing about our shake-up. I drank coffee—a superfood—to get through the event.

In the 21st century, I still enjoy the kitchen during quake swarms and whiteouts. I will cook a healthful entree with fresh spices, herbs, and even java. Chefs use coffee as a secret ingredient in many entrees because it adds flavor. There are delicious recipes in this section, from Slow Roast Shoulder of Lamb with Coffee and Cumin to Prawn Mole, that'll win you over as well as family and friends whether your world is calm or unstable due to Earth's changes.

Coffee Chili
Coffee Pork Chops
Italian Roast Cornish Game Hens with Stuffing
Java-Style Stuffed Bell Peppers
Prawn Mole
Slow Roast Shoulder of Lamb with Coffee and Cumin
Thai Coffee Spiced Chicken Sates
Veggie Lasagna with Coffee Sauce

Coffee Chili

❖ ❖ ❖

1 cup dried red beans
1 cup extra-strength coffee
2 tablespoons vegetable oil
½ cup chopped onion
3 cloves garlic, finely chopped
2 pounds top sirloin steak, cut
   into ½-inch cubes
1½ tablespoons chili powder
1 teaspoon dried oregano
1 teaspoon ground cumin

1 teaspoon dried thyme
1 teaspoon freshly ground pepper
1 can (14½ ounces) tomato puree
   or crushed peeled tomatoes to
   taste
1 cup beef broth
Salt to taste
Sour cream for garnish
Grated cheese for garnish
Cilantro sprigs for garnish

In a mixing bowl, cover the red beans with ¾ cup coffee. Soak overnight. In a deep casserole, heat 1 tablespoon of oil and sauté the onion and garlic over medium heat until soft, about 10 minutes. Set them to one side, add the remaining tablespoon of oil, and brown the steak cubes.

Add the remaining ¼ cup of coffee, spices, and tomato puree or tomatoes to the casserole. Bring to boil, stir well, allow to simmer for 10 minutes. Add the beef broth and the drained beans to the casserole and bring to a boil over medium heat. Reduce the heat and simmer for 1 hour. Season with salt. To serve, ladle the chili into individual bowls and top with the sour cream, grated cheese, and sprigs of cilantro. Serves 4 to 6.

(*Courtesy:* The Roast and Post Coffee Company.)

Coffee Pork Chops

❖ ❖ ❖

6 pork chops
3 tablespoons olive oil
2 mashed cloves garlic
2 teaspoons parsley
150 ml red wine
150 ml strong, black coffee

3 teaspoons honey
Salt and black pepper, freshly
   ground
Juice and grated pulp of a lemon
   or lime

Put the chops inside a large, but low stewpan. Mix the remaining ingredients and drop them all onto the chops. Let it marinate overnight, stirring every now and then. Remove the chops from the stewpan, put them under the grill, and turn them over until uniformly browned. Put them again into the stewpan and bake in a preheated oven at 350°F for 30 minutes. Remove the chops, and skim the fat off the gravy. Serve with rice. Serves 6.

(*Courtesy:* The Roast and Post Coffee Company.)

Italian Roast Cornish Game Hens with Stuffing

❖ ❖ ❖

1⅛ cups butter
2 tablespoons honey (orange sage)
2 premium all-natural Cornish hens

Pepper and ginger to taste
¼ cup Italian Roast coffee, brewed

In a saucepan, melt butter and stir in honey. Wash hens. Place in baking dish. Season hens. Bake at 350°F for one hour and a half or till cooked. Baste periodically with honey butter. Cover with foil the last 10 to 15 minutes. (Use a meat thermometer and when it reads 180 degrees the hens are done.) Serves 4.

CRAN-APPLE NUT STUFFING
½ cup European-style butter
1 diced Fuji apple
⅔ cup fresh whole cranberries

¾–1 cup chopped celery
½ cup chopped walnuts
1 package seasoned stuffing

In a frying pan, melt butter and sauté fruit, celery, and nuts. Add mixture to seasoned stuffing. Stir well. Put into a glass baking dish; pop into oven at 350°F for about an hour. Spoon next to hens. Serves 6 to 8.

Java-Style Stuffed Bell Peppers

❖ ❖ ❖

1 medium onion, minced
1/3 cup extra virgin olive oil
1/2 pound lean ground beef
1/2 pound lean ground pork
6 red bell peppers
1/2 teaspoon black pepper
1/2 teaspoon salt (or to taste)
1/4 teaspoon curry

1/2 cup raisins
1 cup prepared coffee
1/4 cup quick-cooking oatmeal
2 cups cooked rice
1 egg
1/4 cup pine nuts
3 tablespoons bread crumbs

In skillet, cook onion in olive oil for one minute. Add beef and pork; cook until lightly browned. Cut off stem ends of peppers; scoop out white membrane and seeds. Combine all ingredients (except bread crumbs). Cook until liquid is absorbed.

Stuff peppers; sprinkle with bread crumbs. Place in baking pan, cover with foil, and bake 15 minutes at 350°F. Remove foil; bake 15 to 20 minutes more or until peppers are fork tender. Serves 6.

(*Courtesy:* Gemma Sanita Sciabica.)

Prawn Mole

❖ ❖ ❖

30 large prawns (about 2 pounds), shelled
2 bottles beer
1 tablespoon red pepper flakes
1 ounce dried New Mexico chili pods
3 ounces dried mild pasilla chili pods
2 cups double-strength coffee, hot
1 1/2 tablespoons ground coffee
1 tablespoon dried oregano
6 whole cloves
1 1/2 teaspoons ground cinnamon
6 whole allspice

1 teaspoon dried thyme
2 tablespoons grated bitter chocolate
1 tablespoon vegetable oil
1 large onion, chopped
4 large garlic cloves, chopped
1/2 cup golden raisins
3 medium-ripe tomatoes, cut in half
1/4 cup cashews
1/2 cup blanched almonds
Ripe honeydew melon wedges for garnish
Mint for garnish

Place the prawns, beer, and pepper flakes in a non-metallic bowl. Cover and marinate in the refrigerator for several hours. Using kitchen scissors, cut the stems of the chili pods. Open the pods, take out any of the white veins, and reserve the seeds. Place the cleaned pods on a baking sheet and warm in a preheated oven at 300°F for 5 minutes. (Watch the pods carefully so they don't scorch.) Soak the warmed chili pods in 1 1/2 cups hot coffee for 20 minutes.

In a dry frying pan, toast the chili seeds over medium heat for 3 to 5 minutes, shaking the pan to brown the seeds evenly. Place the toasted seeds, ground coffee, spices, and chocolate into a spice grinder or blender and process until all the pieces are finely ground. Reserve.

Heat the oil in a skillet and sauté the chopped onion and garlic for five minutes until translucent. Soak the raisins in the remaining 1/2 cup coffee for 10 minutes. Drain and reserve coffee. Place halved tomatoes, cut side down, on a foil-lined baking sheet and place 6 inches from the heat until the tomato skins bubble slightly and blacken.

In a food processor, whirl the cashews and almonds until finely ground. Add the onion, garlic, tomatoes and raisins. Drain and coarsely chop the reserved chili pods and place in processor. Process thoroughly. Add the coffee-spice mixture and process until combined. This is your mole. (The mole should be moist and thick, resembling oatmeal in texture. Add reserved coffee, a tablespoon at a time, if too dry.) Place the mole in large enamel pot and bring to boil over medium heat. Simmer for 5 minutes, stirring the bottom constantly to keep from scorching the mole. Drain the prawns from the marinade. Place the prawns in the mole sauce and cook over medium heat for 7 minutes, or until just pink and coated with sauce. To serve, place 3 prawns on each plate. Accompany with a small bowl of warmed mole and melon wedges on the side. Garnish with mint. Makes 4 main dishes.

(*Courtesy:* The Roast and Post Coffee Company.)

Slow Roast Shoulder of Lamb with Coffee and Cumin

❖ ❖ ❖

4 tablespoons Turkish coffee

4 tablespoons sesame seeds (toasted)

3 small chilies

2 tablespoons ground cumin

6 cloves garlic

2 fluid ounces pernod

1 shoulder of lamb (blade bone removed)

18 ounces cherry tomatoes

½ pint white wine

4 tablespoons coriander

Combine the first 6 ingredients to a paste. Take the lamb and pierce it all over with a skewer and then rub the paste all over so as to get some of the paste into the holes. Then take a roasting pan and put the tomatoes and wine into the bottom and place the lamb on top, season with sea salt, and transfer to the oven for about 1½ hours. Baste frequently to avoid burning the paste on the outside of the meat.

To serve, lift the tomatoes onto a serving platter and carve the meat and arrange alongside and then serve with the freshly chopped coriander.

(*Courtesy:* The Roast and Post Coffee Company.)

Thai Coffee Spiced Chicken Sates

❖ ❖ ❖

2 tablespoons ground coffee, regular or decaffeinated

2 tablespoons peanut butter, smooth or chunky

3 cloves minced garlic

1 tablespoon minced fresh ginger root

1 teaspoon crushed red chilies

Canola or peanut oil

¼ cup soy sauce

1 tablespoon light brown sugar

2 tablespoons lime juice

1 tablespoon curry powder

2 boneless, skinless chicken breasts cut into ½-inch-wide strips

24 wooden skewers

Combine all ingredients except the chicken and skewers in a bowl and set aside. Thread the chicken on the wooden skewers and place in a dish with raised sides. Pour the marinade (the combined ingredients) over them, cover, and allow to marinate in the refrigerator for at least 2 hours or overnight.

Grill over coals or a gas grill at a medium heat for 5 minutes per side or until cooked through. Be sure to thoroughly cook the chicken (or pork if you're using it). Serves 6–8. Thai Spiced Chicken Sates are sure to be summer pleasers served with a salad, toasted French bread, and a chilled beverage—like iced coffee!

(*Courtesy*: Chef Steve Petusevsky; National Coffee Association of U.S.A., Inc., Coffee Science Source.)

Veggie Lasagna with Coffee Sauce

❖ ❖ ❖

1 package lasagna noodles, whole
   grain or gourmet
1 package low-fat Monterey Jack
   or cheddar cheese, shredded
2 cups ricotta cheese
1 8-ounce package low-fat
   mozzarella, shredded

½ cup Italian Roast coffee, brewed
24-ounce jar marinara sauce (with
   olive oil, garlic, mushrooms)
2½ cups fresh vegetables (broccoli, zucchini, tomatoes), chopped
Nutmeg and pepper to taste

In a large saucepan, boil pasta al dente. Drain. In a mixing bowl, combine cheeses. Add coffee to marinara sauce. Set aside. Boil vegetables for a few minutes. Add nutmeg and pepper to taste. In a 9-inch-by-13-inch baking dish (I use a rustic red Italian one), layer ingredients: sauces, pasta, vegetables, and cheese. Repeat. The top layer will be sauce topped with mozzarella. Cover with foil to prevent burning the edges of the pasta; remove foil after the first 20 minutes in the oven. Bake at 350°F for 70 minutes until bubbly. Serves 10 to 12.

Desserts

A few years ago, I ended up in Seattle at Pike Place Market (the place Starbucks opened its doors), which has the strong flavor of San Francisco's Fisherman's Wharf. With a double mocha latte from the famed coffee company, I strolled and felt the caffeine buzz that helped me go on the quest for the perfect sweatshirt and key chain with a Brittany, my choice of dog. Enjoying sights of fish, fruit, flowers, and strangers was bliss (it had to be the caffeine fix).

I could have joined people after the book lecture/signing, but there was something special about savoring a day with me and joe, from the first thing in the morning to that afternoon, that made my Washington trip comforting and invigorating.

While gourmet coffee and desserts are perfect for anytime, they're even more decadent during an afternoon coffee break. There are so many types of roasts, blends, and flavored types to pair with quickie foods for snacks. These scrumptious and healthful appetizers will allow you to pamper yourself in a different, exciting place even if you're in the comfort of your own home.

In this section you'll notice that I've included plenty of desserts, because I am a dessert lover. I chose recipes that include common foods of Oldways Mediterranean Diet Pyramid. Naturally, Cappuccino Cookies and Tiramisu will rock your world. Once you begin baking with coffee, it will wake up your palate.

Almond Coffee Cream
Cappuccino Chip–Fruit Bundt Cake
Cappuccino Cookies
Chocolate Carrot Cake with Cappuccino Frosting
Chocolate Ricotta Bundt Cake with Espresso Frosting
Coffee Flan
Easy Mocha Brownie Torte
Espresso Orange Chiffon Squares
Maple Espresso Pudding
Mystery Mocha Cake

Profiterols with Coffee Rum Sauce
Rosemary-Infused Chocolate Fudge Cake
with Chocolate-Tofu Frosting
Tiramisu

Almond Coffee Cream

❖ ❖ ❖

2 teaspoons coffee, finely ground
to a powder
¼ cup skim milk
½ teaspoon salt
2 egg whites
Low-calorie sugar substitute
(equal to 1/4 cup sugar)

⅛ teaspoon almond extract
¼ cup finely chopped almonds
4 ounces non-dairy whipped
topping, thawed

Dissolve coffee in milk and set aside. Add the salt to the egg whites and beat until foamy. Gradually add the sugar substitute and continue to beat until the mixture forms stiff, shiny peaks. Blend in the coffee/milk mixture, almond extract, and chopped almonds. Fold in the dietetic topping. Spoon into individual parfait glasses. Garnish with chopped almonds if desired. Freeze until firm. Serves 6.

(*Courtesy*: National Coffee Association of U.S.A., Inc.)

Cappuccino Chip–Fruit Bundt Cake

❖ ❖ ❖

1 premium yellow cake mix
3 large brown eggs
⅔ cup water
⅔ cup organic 2 percent low-fat
milk
3 tablespoons European-style
butter, melted

1 cup cappuccino chips (King
Arthur)
1 cup dark chocolate chips
Extra virgin olive oil (for greasing
pan)
1 tablespoon whole-wheat flour
(for dusting pan)

GARNISH

Confectioners' sugar

½ cup fresh cherries or strawberries, whole with stems

In a mixing bowl, combine cake mix, eggs, beaten, liquid ingredients, and butter. Stir a few minutes till smooth. Fold in 2 cups of chips. Lightly grease tube pan with butter and dust with flour. Pour in batter and bake at 350°F for about 45 minutes. (Put knife in and if it comes out clean, it's done.) Cool. Use a knife to loosen the cake from the pan and turn over on a plate. Sprinkle sugar on top. Place ½ cup fresh cherries or berries in the middle. Serves 10.

Cappuccino Cookies

❖ ❖ ❖

1¼ cups brown sugar
½ teaspoon salt
3 tablespoons espresso powder
½ teaspoon salt
¼ cup brewed coffee
½ cup Marsala Olive Oil
2 eggs
1 tablespoon corn syrup
1 teaspoon vanilla
1 tablespoon honey

½ teaspoon Danish pastry extract (Watkins)
1 teaspoon baking soda
2¾ cups flour
1 tablespoon cocoa (Dutch)
1 cup cappuccino chips
½ cup mini cinnamon chips
½ cup white chocolate chips or chunks (if desired)
Grated peel of 1 orange

Preheat oven to 375°; grease cookie sheets. In mixing bowl combine dry ingredients; make well in center. Pour in coffee, olive oil, eggs, corn syrup, and flavorings; stir to blend. Add chips; scoop rounded teaspoons of dough onto prepared pans, 2 inches apart. Bake cookies 10 to 14 minutes; do not over bake. Cool on wire rack. Drizzle with melted white chocolate if desired. Cappuccino and cinnamon chips may be purchased from a variety of online candy companies.

(Courtesy: *Baking Sensational Sweets with California Olive Oil*, by Gemma Sanita Sciabica.)

Chocolate Carrot Cake with
Cappuccino Frosting

❖ ❖ ❖

1 cup flour
¾ cup sugar
¼ cup cocoa (Dutch)
1 teaspoon baking soda
1 teaspoon salt
½ teaspoon cinnamon
¼ teaspoon nutmeg

3 tablespoons Marsala Olive Oil
¼ cup orange juice (or milk)
¼ teaspoon vanilla
2 eggs
Grated peel of 1 orange
2 ounces coconut
2½ cups carrots, shredded

In a mixing bowl add dry ingredients. Make well in center. Add olive oil, juice, vanilla, eggs, and peel. Stir until blended. Fold in coconut and carrots well. Pour into greased 8-inch-square baking pan. Bake 30 to 35 minutes in 350-degree oven. Frost.

FROSTING
½ cup cappuccino chips

Remove cake from oven, sprinkle with chips; let stand about 3 to 5 minutes. When chips have melted, spread top completely. Makes 12 to 16 pieces.

(Courtesy: Cooking with California Olive Oil: Treasured Family Recipes, by Gemma Sanita Sciabica.)

Chocolate Ricotta Bundt Cake with Espresso Frosting

❖ ❖ ❖

This chocolate ricotta cake is moist with a nice chocolaty flavor—but not devil's food cake. The nuts add a crunch, and cocoa powder gives an extra chocolate taste. This cake, freshly baked or warmed up in the microwave, is a fine Mediterranean version of a chocolate dessert made with real ingredients. It let me feel like I was a character in the film *Under the Tuscan Sun*. Thanks to my homespun chocolate cake, I transcended to an Italian bistro without leaving the comfort of my cozy cabin.

BUNDT CAKE

2 cups unbleached white whole-wheat flour
⅓ cup unsweetened premium cocoa powder
½ cup granulated sugar
2 teaspoons baking powder
½ cup light brown sugar
2 brown eggs

1 cup ricotta cheese
¼ cup European-style butter
1⅓ cups half-and-half milk
2 tablespoons sour cream
1 cup chocolate chips, 60 percent cacao
1 teaspoon pure vanilla extract

In a medium-sized bowl, combine dry ingredients. Then, add mixture of eggs, cheese, melted butter, half-and-half, sour cream, chocolate chips, and vanilla. Mix well. Pour batter into an 8-by-8-inch square baking dish. Bake at 350°F for about 25 to 30 minutes. Cool.

ESPRESSO FROSTING

2 teaspoons instant espresso powder
4 tablespoons European-style butter, melted

2½ cups confectioners' sugar
1 teaspoon pure vanilla extract
½ cup almonds, sliced
1 tablespoon cocoa powder

In a bowl, mix coffee, butter, and sugar to the consistency preferred. Add vanilla and cocoa powder. Spread with a spatula on top of cake. Sprinkle with nuts. Slice cake into squares. Place on simple plate and dust with cocoa powder. Serves 9 to 12.

Coffee Flan

❖ ❖ ❖

¾ cup sugar
1 cup brewed Chock full o'Nuts
  coffee
⅛ teaspoon salt
1 teaspoon vanilla

5 large eggs
3¾ cups whole milk
1 (14-ounce) can sweetened con-
  densed milk (1¼ cups)

Put oven rack in middle position and preheat oven to 350°F. Cook sugar in a dry small heavy saucepan over moderate heat until it begins to melt. Continue to cook, stirring occasionally with a fork, until sugar melts into a golden caramel. Immediately pour into a 9-inch round ceramic or glass baking dish or metal cake pan (1 inch deep) and tilt dish to coat bottom. Cool until hardened, 10 to 15 minutes.

Over medium-low heat, reduce the coffee down to ⅓ cup of liquid. Blend this with the remaining ingredients until smooth. Pour this custard through a fine-mesh sieve over caramel in dish, then transfer dish to a 17-by-11-inch roasting pan lined with a kitchen towel. Cover dish loosely with a piece of foil, then pour enough boiling-hot water into roasting pan to reach 1 inch up side of dish. Bake until custard is set but still wobbly in center when gently shaken and a knife inserted in center comes out clean, 1 to 1⅓ hours. Transfer dish to a rack to cool, 40 minutes. Chill flan, covered, at least 8 hours.

(*Courtesy*: Chock full o'Nuts.)

Easy Mocha Brownie Torte

❖ ❖ ❖

8 ounces butter
4 ounces unsweetened cooking
  chocolate, broken into pieces
4 eggs
1 teaspoon vanilla extract
15 ounces sugar

4½ ounces flour
4 ounces finely chopped pecans
Mocha Cream Filling (recipe
  follows)
Semi-Sweet Glaze (recipe follows)

Line bottom and sides of two 9-inch round pans with foil; grease foil. Melt butter and unsweetened chocolate. Cool 5 minutes. In large bowl, beat eggs and vanilla until foamy. Gradually add sugar, beating well. Blend in chocolate mixture; fold in flour and pecans until blended. Spread half the mixture into each prepared pan. Bake 20 to 25 minutes at 350°F or until wooden pick inserted in center comes out clean. Cool 5 minutes; using foil, remove from pans to wire racks. Peel off foil and cool completely. Place one layer on serving plate; spread with Mocha Cream Filling. Glaze second with Semi-Sweet Glaze. Cover; refrigerate until ready to serve. To serve, gently place glazed layer on top of mocha filling layer. Refrigerate leftover torte. Serves 10 to 12.

Mocha Cream Filling

Reserve 2 tablespoons from 8 fluid ounces cold whipping cream for glaze. In small bowl, place remaining whipping cream, 3 tablespoons powdered sugar, and 2 teaspoons powdered instant coffee. Beat until stiff.

Semi-Sweet Glaze

Melt 3 ounces semi-sweet cooking chocolate and reserved whipping cream together, just until chocolate is melted and mixture is smooth when stirred.

(*Courtesy*: The Roast and Post Coffee Company.)

Espresso Orange Chiffon Squares

❖ ❖ ❖

4 eggs separated (room temperature)
1⅓ cups sugar
1¾ cups flour
2 tablespoons espresso instant
    coffee powder
½ teaspoon salt

3 teaspoons baking powder
⅔ cup milk, non-fat
3 tablespoons Marsala Olive Oil
½ teaspoon almond extract
1 teaspoon vanilla
Grated peel of 1 orange

Lightly grease and flour a 9-by-13-inch cake pan. In a large mixing bowl add egg whites; beat until frothy. Add 1/2 cup sugar; beat until whites hold stiff peaks. In another bowl add remaining sugar, flour, coffee powder, salt, and baking powder. Make a well in center, add yolks, milk, oil, and flavorings; stir until smooth. Pour batter over egg whites; fold gently until well blended. Pour batter into prepared pan.

Bake in 350-degree oven for 35 to 40 minutes or until cake springs back when lightly pressed with fingertip on center. Cool on cake rack, turn out onto serving plate, and cut cake into 2 layers.

FILLING

1 5-ounce package chocolate or
    vanilla pudding

1 cup raspberry, blackberry or
    apricot jam

Cook pudding according to directions on package, using ½ cup less milk; cool. Cover bottom layer of cake evenly with raspberry jam. Top with chocolate pudding evenly.

TOPPING

½ pint whipping cream
1 tablespoon rum or Irish Cream
    liqueur
½ cup confectioners' sugar
2 teaspoons espresso instant coffee
    powder

½ cup pistachios or hazelnuts
    chopped fine
Cream whipped with coffee powder,
    rum, and sugar until still

Cover bottom layer of cake with second layer; frost with espresso whipped cream. Sprinkle with nuts. Cut into 20 to 24 squares. Serves about 20 to 24.

(*Courtesy:* Gemma Sanita Sciabica, *Baking with California Olive Oil: Dolci and Biscotti Recipes.*)

Maple Espresso Pudding

❖ ❖ ❖

2¼ ounces, plus ½ tablespoon
   dark brown sugar
2 tablespoons cornstarch
Pinch of salt
1 cup whole milk
1½ cups heavy cream

1 tablespoon espresso coffee
1 ounce maple syrup
2 tablespoons unsalted butter, cut
   into bits
1¼ teaspoons pure vanilla extract

Whisk together brown sugar, cornstarch, and pinch of salt in a heavy medium saucepan, then whisk in milk, 1 cup heavy cream, espresso coffee, and maple syrup. Bring to boil over medium heat, whisking frequently, then boil, whisking, 1 minute. Remove from heat and whisk in butter and 1 teaspoon vanilla. Pour into a bowl, then cover surface with buttered wax paper and chill until cold, at least 1½ hours. Whip remaining ½ cup heavy cream, ½ tablespoon sugar, and ¼ teaspoon vanilla until medium peaks. Fold into above until consistency is smooth. Serves 2.

(*Courtesy*: Pastry Sous Janine Fong, Claremont Hotel Club & Spa.)

Mystery Mocha Cake

❖ ❖ ❖

The only mysterious thing about this cake is how it can be so delicious and still contain virtually no fat. Looking at this deep, almost black chocolate cake, cushioned in a velvety fudge sauce, you'll think, "No way. No way is this cake low calorie." But, at 124 calories a serving (not including the whipped cream/ice cream you'll be dying to add) it won't push your calorie count for the day into the stratosphere.

CAKE
¾ cup (5¼ ounces) granulated
   sugar
1 cup (4¼ ounces) King Arthur
   unbleached all-purpose or
   white whole wheat flour

2 teaspoons baking powder
¼ teaspoon salt
¼ cup (¾ ounce) low-fat cocoa
¾ cup (6 ounces) skim milk
2 teaspoons vanilla

SAUCE

½ cup (3¼ ounces) brown sugar,
    packed
½ cup (3½ ounces) granulated
    sugar

¾ ounce low-fat cocoa
1 cup (8 ounces) double-strength
    coffee, room temperature

CAKE

Preheat the oven to 350°F. Lightly grease an 8-by-8-inch baking pan. In a large mixing bowl, stir together sugar, flour, baking powder, salt, and cocoa. Add the milk and vanilla; beat till smooth. Pour the batter into a lightly greased 8-by-8-inch pan.

SAUCE

In a small bowl, mix together the white and brown sugars and cocoa. Sprinkle evenly over the batter in the pan. Pour the coffee over all. This may look kind of strange and messy, but never fear; everything will turn out fine.

Bake the cake for 40 minutes, or until the top springs back when pressed gently. Remove from the oven and cool on a wire rack. This cake is best enjoyed warm, between half an hour and an hour after you've taken it out of the oven. Yield: 1 cake, sixteen 2-by-2-inch servings.

(*Courtesy:* King Arthur Flour.)

Profiterols with Coffee Rum Sauce

❖ ❖ ❖

THE PUFFS

2 cups boiling water
⅛ teaspoon salt
1 cup butter

2 cups all-purpose flour
8 eggs

Preheat oven to 400°F. Bring the water to a boil in a medium-sized saucepan. Add salt and butter and stir until the butter has melted. Reduce the heat. Add the flour and beat the mixture until it comes away from the side of the pan and forms a smooth ball in the center. Remove from heat and add eggs, one at a time, beating well. Using a dessert spoon, shape the puffs and place them on a lightly greased cookie sheet. Bake at 400°F for 8 minutes, then reduce heat to 350°F and bake for an additional 10 to 12 minutes. Remove puffs from the oven and let cool. Slice off the top of each puff and fill the cavity with cream. Arrange the puffs in the shape of a pyramid. Pour Coffee Rum Sauce over them and serve. Serves 8.

THE CREAM

4 tablespoons strong cold coffee   Sugar to taste
2 cups heavy cream, whipped

Slowly add the cold coffee to the whipped cream, and fold in well. Sweeten to taste.

COFFEE RUM SAUCE

1 cup sugar   3 tablespoons cold coffee
1½ cups (12 ounces) strong coffee   2 tablespoons butter
2 tablespoons cornstarch   2 tablespoons rum

Slowly melt sugar in a saucepan over low heat, stirring constantly. Gradually add strong coffee, continuing to stir constantly until the sugar is completely dissolved. In a small bowl stir the cornstarch into the cold coffee and combine with heated mixture. Cook combined ingredients until they boil and thicken. Remove from the heat. Add butter and rum. Stir until butter melts. Let cool to room temperature.

(*Courtesy:* Coffee Science Source.)

Rosemary-Infused Chocolate Fudge Cake with Chocolate-Tofu Frosting

❖ ❖ ❖

Coffee infused with fresh rosemary and cocoa gives this luscious fudge cake its distinctive flavor.

FOR THE CAKE

*Vegetable oil in a spray bottle, or
  1 teaspoon vegetable oil
4 sprigs fresh rosemary
½ cup hot, strong, freshly brewed
  coffee
1 teaspoon teaspoon Kahlúa or
  coffee brandy (optional)
1 large ripe banana*

*½ cup packed brown sugar
1 cup unbleached flour, sifted
¾ cup cocoa powder, sifted
1 teaspoon baking powder
½ teaspoon baking soda
¼ teaspoon ground cinnamon
4 egg whites, at room temperature
¼ teaspoon kosher salt*

FOR THE FROSTING

*½ cup firm silken tofu, drained
2 tablespoons pure maple syrup
2 tablespoons cocoa powder, sifted*

*2 tablespoons commercial chocolate-
  flavored soy milk*

Preheat the oven to 375°F. Spray or grease a 6-inch round baking pan with vegetable oil; set aside.

Steep the rosemary sprigs in the hot coffee for 15 minutes. Remove the sprigs; set aside and let cool.

Pour the cooled rosemary-infused coffee, vanilla extract, and Kahlúa or coffee brandy, if using, into a blender or food processor fitted with a metal blade. Add the banana; process until smooth. Transfer to a mixing bowl and stir in the brown sugar.

In another large mixing bowl, combine the flour, cocoa powder, baking powder, baking soda, and cinnamon. Stir in the mixture of coffee, banana, and brown sugar; mix well.

Using an eggbeater or electric mixer fitted with a whip, beat the egg whites and salt at high speed until they form soft peaks. Gently fold the whipped egg whites into the batter until they are fully incorporated. Pour into the prepared pan; bake for 30 to 35 minutes, or until toothpick inserted into the center of the cake comes out clean. Remove from the oven, turn out onto a rack, and let cool for about 20 minutes.

Meanwhile, make the frosting by combining the tofu, maple syrup, cocoa powder, and soy milk in a wide-based blender or a food processor fitted with a metal blade; process until smooth, then transfer to a bowl.

When the cake has cooled completely, use a spatula to frost the top and sides of the cake. Makes 1 (6-inch) round cake. Serves 6.

(Reprinted with permission from *The Golden Door Cooks Light & Easy* by Chef Michel Stroot, published by Gibbs Smith, © 2003.)

Tiramisu

❖ ❖ ❖

3 egg yolks
¼ cup sugar
1¼ cups coffee liqueur (Kahlúa)
1 tablespoon espresso coffee powder
2 cups mascarpone cheese, room temperature

1 egg white, whipped
1 cup cream, whipped
1 sponge sheet cake, sliced into ladyfinger size pieces
2 tablespoons Dutch cocoa powder

In top of double broiler, beat egg yolks and sugar. Add ¼ cup Kahlúa and beat over simmering heat, until mixture begins to thicken; let cool. Stir coffee powder into mascarpone. Beat egg white until stiff. Fold egg white into mascarpone mixture. Whip cream until still. Dip sponge cake pieces into remaining Kahlúa; arrange in a single layer in bottom of a deep straight-sided serving bowl.

Cover cake pieces with ½ of the mascarpone mixture, ½ of the egg yolk mixture, then ½ of the cream. Repeat the layers with sponge pieces dipped into Kahlúa, mascarpone mixture, and egg yolk mixture, finishing with the cream. Dust top with cocoa powder. Refrigerate until ready to serve. Serves 8.

(*Courtesy:* Gemma Sanita Sciabica, *Baking with California Olive Oil: Dolci and Biscotti Recipes.*)

Candy

During the summer at Lake Tahoe it reminds me of Stephen King's *The Langoliers*. When tourists invade our town my stress level soars. One Sunday afternoon, I did hit escape to the local outdoor pool and swam laps like a mermaid. Back home I could hear tourists' dogs barking, kids and adults laughing, and concert music bellowing. To cope, I ended up turning to sweet, hard coffee candy, which I got from Oh! Nuts, an online store.

I don't know if it's the caffeine, sugar, or crunchy texture—or combo—but it and an iced coffee got me through the invasion and helped me to focus while working in Coffee World day and night, much like my college days when I pulled all-nighters for the school newspaper. Candy recipes that you can make, such as Kahlúa Coffee Fudge, are easy to make and available year-round.

Cappuccino Blocks
Kahlúa Creamy Fudge

Cappuccino Blocks

❖ ❖ ❖

Swirl these soft, candy-like blocks into a mug of hot milk and enjoy luscious espresso steamers.

1 cup heavy cream, divided
1 tablespoon espresso powder
2 tablespoons corn syrup
¼ teaspoon salt
1 cup sugar
1 tablespoon (½ ounce) vanilla
bean or vanilla extract

2 cups chopped white chocolate
1 tablespoon cocoa, natural or
Dutch-process
½ teaspoon espresso powder
Wooden sticks or stir sticks

Line an 8-by-8-inch pan with parchment or aluminum foil, and spray lightly with non-stick baking spray. Place ½ cup cream in a medium saucepan. Add the espresso powder, corn syrup, salt, and sugar. Stir over medium heat until the espresso powder and sugar are dissolved and the mixture begins to boil. Cover the pan and let boil for 3 minutes. Uncover the pan, and check the temperature; it should be 235 to 240°F (soft ball stage). If it is, remove from heat; otherwise let it boil for a minute or two more. Once the mixture reaches 235 to 240°F, add the vanilla. Be careful; it will splash and splutter when it hits the hot liquid. Set the mixture aside for about 10 minutes to cool. Meanwhile, place the remaining ½ cup cream into a saucepan. Heat until it's just beginning to steam. Remove from the heat, and add the white chocolate. Let sit for about 5 minutes to melt. Then whisk vigorously until the mixture is shiny and smooth. Add the sugar mixture to the chocolate mixture; stir to combine. Combine the cocoa and ½ teaspoon espresso, and sprinkle the chocolate with some of the mixture. Refrigerate for at least 4 hours to set. Turn the chocolate out of the pan and flip it over; sprinkle with the remaining cocoa/espresso powder blend. Cut into cubes. Stack two or three on a wooden stick. Roll in cocoa, or whatever you sprinkled on the top and bottom. Wrap in wax paper, parchment, or plastic wrap to store. Yield about 64 blocks, 21 servings.

(*Courtesy:* King Arthur Flour.)

Kahlúa Creamy Fudge

❖ ❖ ❖

1⅓ *cups granulated sugar*
1 *7-ounce jar marshmallow crème*
⅔ *cup evaporated milk*
¼ *cup butter*
¼ *cup Kahlúa*

¼ *teaspoon salt*
2 *cups semi-sweet chocolate pieces*
1 *cup milk chocolate pieces*
⅔ *cup chopped nuts*
1 *teaspoon vanilla*

Line 8-inch square baking tray with foil. In a 2-quart saucepan, combine sugar, marshmallow crème, milk, butter, Kahlúa, and salt. Bring to a rapid boil, stirring constantly for 5 minutes. Remove from heat; add all chocolate. Stir until melted. Add nuts and vanilla. Turn into the prepared baking tray. Refrigerate until firm. To serve, cut in squares. Makes about 2¾ pounds.

(*Courtesy:* The Roast and Post Coffee Company.)

Beverages

On day three of the power outage at Tahoe (the one I mentioned earlier and how I turned to my lifesaver—instant coffee) the electricity was back on when I awoke in the early morning. To celebrate life again as I knew it, I reunited with Mr. Coffee and savored not one but two cups of hot French Vanilla Roast. I missed organic low-fat milk—but I sprinkled cinnamon on top and anticipated a big grocery shopping trip that day to get milk (from half-and-half to organic chocolate milk)—and whipped cream because it was a time to savor the joys of electricity and cold milk and gourmet coffee.

But I didn't go through coffee withdrawal, thanks to instant coffee. Going without power was bad enough. I was plugged in and I survived with joe. Once you get used to brewed coffee, going back to the quickie stuff is a challenge. These coffee recipes, especially the hot drinks, from a chilled Coffee Alexander to steamy Pumpkin Spice Latte, will remind you just how special specialty coffee drinks can be.

Cold Drinks:
Chocolate Intemperance
Coffee Alexander
Iced Chocolate Mochaccino
Sassy Sodas

Hot Drinks:
Brown Sugar Caramel Latte
Café Mexicano
Eggnog Latte
Pumpkin Spice Latte

Chocolate Intemperance

❖ ❖ ❖

This recipe makes a thick, rich, cold chocolate drink that's delicious served as is, or blended with ice to make a chocolate smoothie.

½ cup Dutch-process cocoa
1 cup sugar
3 tablespoons Instant ClearJel or
  cornstarch
¼ teaspoon salt
1 cup water

1 tablespoon vanilla or espresso
  powder or 1 teaspoon cinnamon
  (all optional)
2 cups milk or cream
1 cup chopped semi-sweet or bittersweet chocolate

In a medium saucepan, whisk together the cocoa, sugar, ClearJel or cornstarch, and salt. Slowly whisk in the water, then the flavoring of your choice and the milk or cream. Bring to a boil over medium heat, whisking constantly. Remove from the heat and stir in the chocolate, whisking till chocolate melts. Pour into a bowl, and stir occasionally as it cools, to prevent a skin from forming. Pour into a jar or other storage container, and lay a piece of plastic wrap on the surface of the chocolate, again to prevent a skin from forming. Store in the refrigerator for up to a week. Yield: 1½ cups chocolate base.

Serve as is, in very small glasses; it's thick and rich. To make one frozen smoothie, place ⅓ cup chocolate base in a blender. Add about 1 cup ice cubes (and 1 ounce of the spirit of your choice, if desired), and blend till smooth. Alternatively, blend with chunks of banana, or a scoop of ice cream.

Feeling intemperate? Add vodka and coffee liqueur to ⅓ cup chocolate for the best sweet martini ever! To rim glass with cinnamon sugar, mix 1 teaspoon cinnamon with 2 tablespoons sparkling sugar and 1 tablespoon granulated sugar. Wipe the edge of the glass with a wet cloth, then dip it into the sugar mixture.

(*Courtesy:* King Arthur Flour.)

Coffee Alexander

❖ ❖ ❖

1 cup cold strong coffee
2 ounces brandy or cognac

1 cup coffee ice cream

Pour all ingredients into a blender and blend until smooth and creamy. Serve in champagne or wine glasses. Garnish each with a coffee bean. Serves 2.

(*Courtesy*: National Coffee Association of U.S.A., Inc.)

Iced Chocolate Mochaccino

❖ ❖ ❖

½ cup MarieBelle's Aztec Iced
  Chocolate mix

One shot espresso
Two cups of ice

Pour ½ cup MarieBelle Aztec Iced Chocolate mix into a pot. Pour in a hot shot of espresso and stir in thoroughly until the mixture has a sauce-like texture. Add mixture to a blender with two cups of ice cubes and blend 30–40 seconds. Serve.

(*Courtesy*: MarieBelle.)

Sassy Sodas

❖ ❖ ❖

1 pint coffee ice cream
½ cup light rum
2 tablespoons ground Chock
  full o'Nuts 100% Colombian
  coffee

4 to 6 scoops vanilla ice cream
Cocoa powder

Spoon coffee ice cream into blender container. Add rum and coffee that has been finely ground to a powdery texture. Blend on high speed until creamy smooth. Pour into tall glasses, adding a scoop of vanilla ice cream to each glass. Sprinkle lightly with cocoa powder. Serve with long-handled spoons and soda straws.

(*Courtesy:* Chock full o'Nuts.)

Brown Sugar Caramel Latte

❖ ❖ ❖

1 tablespoon brown sugar
¼ cup half-and-half

¾ cup fresh, black coffee
1 tablespoon caramel sauce

Begin by mixing your brown sugar with the half-and-half until it is completely dissolved. Use the steamer on your espresso machine to froth the half-and-half and brown sugar until hot. Pour your coffee into a large mug, and mix in the caramel sauce completely. Next, pour in the half-and-half mixture, and serve immediately for a sweet and delicious cup of joe!

(*Courtesy:* The Coffee Bump.)

Café Mexicano

❖ ❖ ❖

8 cups water
⅓ cup firm brown sugar
2 whole cloves
1 cinnamon stick
8 ounces whipping cream

1 ounce unsweetened baking
   chocolate
1 cup Chock full o'Nuts Original
   ground coffee
1 teaspoon vanilla

In a medium saucepan over medium-high heat, bring water to a boil. Stir in brown sugar, cloves, and cinnamon stick (broken in half). Reduce heat and simmer for 15 minutes. While mixture simmers, whip cream to soft peaks. Hold in refrigerator. Remove brown sugar/spice mixture from heat; stir in chocolate until melted. Add ground coffee, cover, and let stand 5 minutes. Stir in vanilla. Strain mixture through cheesecloth or a coffee filter. Serve immediately in coffee mugs garnished with whipped cream. Serves 8.

(*Courtesy:* Chock full o'Nuts.)

Eggnog Latte

❖ ❖ ❖

1 tablespoon instant coffee ½ *cup eggnog*
½ *cup boiling water* *Nutmeg*

This recipe is incredibly easy to whip up for a delicious holiday indulgence! Start out by mixing the instant coffee with boiling water, and stir well to dissolve. Stir in the eggnog, and simply sprinkle with a dash of nutmeg to enjoy. Eggnog is a fantastic holiday drink to use as an addition to your coffee beverage, and since this recipe uses instant coffee, you can easily whip it up on your way to work or for an after-dinner drink.

(*Courtesy*: The Coffee Bump.)

Pumpkin Spice Latte

❖ ❖ ❖

Craving a hot pumpkin latte rather than a regular cup of joe? It's so easy to make it yourself. (Flavored pumpkin spice coffee is good, too.) In an 8-ounce mug, combine ½ cup brewed coffee (caramel flavored is yummy) with ½ cup organic low-fat half-and-half. Add 1 teaspoon pumpkin pie filling and 1 teaspoon pumpkin pie spice, whisk or blend. Heat up mixture in microwave. Top with a dollop of whipped cream.

(*Courtesy*: The Coffee Bump.)

A Final Jolt

If this is coffee, please bring me some tea,
if this is tea, please bring me coffee.
—Abraham Lincoln[2]

These days, I'm no longer in my green coffee plant stage. I'm a middle-aged semi-wannabe coffee snob who recalls her first bite of a coffee ice-cream cone. I confess that I do coffee to wake up and sometimes stay up—but my world of coffee is so much more. I've drunk it steaming hot and iced cold, black and bitter and brown and creamy with milk. I stay clear of adding sugar, cream, and no-cal sweeteners. I sweeten it with premium ice cream, dark chocolate shavings, cinnamon, and nutmeg. I've steamed it to make café lattes and café mochas. I cook and bake with it—all flavors, all roasts.

Fresh beans and a blade grinder (I vow to get a burr one to achieve even coffee grounds) are part of my daily ritual. An efficient and eco-friendly coffee pod brewer and pods are in my vocabulary. Last week I turned to making a batch of scones and I used espresso powder in the batter and for the frosting. Coffee has a place in my life to death do us part. (I hope they have coffee, swimming pools, dogs and cats in heaven.)

THE COFFEE TREE PHILOSOPHY

Still, today in the 21st century there are doctors, nutritionists, and maybe even you who believe coffee is an only wake-up beverage, nothing more. Brew one cup of gourmet coffee for a lift and please go back to chapter 1 and reread my words to get that coffee has healing powers—it truly is nature's miracle brew.

Coffee Tree Tip 1: Tune into your body, mind, and spirit like a mature tree that has been on earth for years. If you feel unbalanced turn to coffee to help you get back on an even keel.

Coffee Tree Tip 2: Drinking coffee and not eating a wholesome diet isn't the deal for getting healing powers. Think balance and moderation, much like a coffee tree that has been nourished by its workers. Combine good food and good coffee to have the best of both worlds.

Coffee Tree Tip 3: Stay productive. Finding out why you're on this planet will help you feel your best. Then, when you drink coffee you can continue to feed your purpose and sense of self.

Coffee Tree Tip 4: Take care of yourself and listen to your gut instincts. Like a tree, you know when you're not being nurtured. Nurture you so you can nurture others.

So, as I end my journey in Coffee World, I feel like the coffee tree and I are kindred spirits. And it's coffee that took me to a magical mystery place that was foreign but now is familiar. Like a fifty-something coffee tree I am here on earth to provide healing powers to God's creatures, big and small.

And nowadays, I get it when people say, "More coffee, please." But I add, "I'd like a cup of organic coffee from Brazil or Guatemala. If you don't have it, I'll take a nutty or chocolaty flavored 100 percent Colombian. If you have low-fat organic milk, please add ¼ cup to a 12-ounce mug." That would be my perfect beverage in the land of coffee.

PART 9

COFFEE
RESOURCES

Where Can You Buy Coffee?

As coffee continues to be touted for its healing powers, quality coffee for the health-conscious is becoming more in demand. Currently, a wide world of coffees can be bought in supermarkets, specialty stores, and health food stores, as well as over the Internet.

Here is a list of coffees and coffee products, from organic and all-natural to gourmet brands. If you're interested in buying any of these popular coffees or coffee-related items, just contact the coffee company directly for the locations of stores nearest you.

COFFEE BEAUTY PRODUCTS

Body Coffee
www.bodycoffee.com

Natural body care and spa products.

Juara
www.juaraskincare.com

Makers of an invigorating coffee body scrub made with fresh Indonesian coffee beans to exfoliate and cleanse.

COFFEE RETAILERS/ROASTERS

Alpen Sierra Coffee Roasting Company
800-531-1405; 775-783-7263
www.alpensierracoffee.com

A small but noteworthy roaster, offering an array of coffees, including Hawaiian Hazelnut.

Coffees of Hawaii
P.O. Box 37
1630 Farrington Avenue
Kualapuu, HI 96757
877-322-3276
www.coffeesofhawaii.com

A variety of Hawaiian coffees, including the best-seller Muleskinner and Kona, Island Blends, and unroasted beans.

Coffee, Tea & Spice
54352 430th Avenue
Talihina, OK 74571
866-692-1415; 918-567-5342
www.coffeecoffee.com

Emmie & Ellie's Online Coffee Shop
800-344-2739
www.coffee.org

Incredible products galore, from brand-name coffee products—including coffees, coffee brewers, and pods—to gourmet coffee cakes and much more.

Gillies Coffee Company
Brooklyn, NY
718-499-7766; 800-344-5526
www.gilliescoffee.com

Gillies Coffee, "the oldest coffee merchant in America," is a renowned specialty roaster manufacturing estate and micro-lot coffees, origins, blends, and espresso, in addition to flavored coffees.

Jelks Gourmet Coffee Roasters
P.O. Box 8667
Shreveport, LA 71148
800-235-7361
www.jelks-coffee.com

Awesome flavored coffees that'll impress you, your family, and friends.

Massimo Zanetti Beverage USA, Inc.
200 Port Centre Parkway
Portsmouth, VA 23704
Consumer line: 888-246-2598; business line: 757-215-7300
www.mzb-usa.com
www.chockfullonuts.com
www.hillsbros.com

Maui Oma Coffee Roasting Company
296 Alamaha Street, #J
Kahului, Hawaii 96732
800-900-9820; 808-871-8664
www.hawaiicoffee.net

A variety of Hawaiian coffees, including Maui and Kona coffees.

Starbucks Coffee Company
Seattle, WA
800-STARBUC (800-782-7282)
www.starbucks.com

Opening its doors back in 1971, today Starbucks is a household name, boasting more than 17,000 stores in 55 countries around the globe.

The Roast and Post Coffee Company
www.realcoffee.co.uk

White Coffee Corporation
18-35 38th Street (Steinway Place)
Long Island City, NY 11105
800-221-0140
www.whitecoffee.com

White Coffee Corporation is a third-generation family-owned coffee importing and roasting business in operation since 1939. White Coffee is proud to feature products that are certified "organic" by Quality Insurance International and "fair trade" by Fair Trade USA.

Zecuppa Coffee, LLC
P.O. Box 55
Tracyton, WA 98393
360-698-0618
www.zecuppa.com

Zecuppa Coffee is a specialty coffee roaster and bulk supplier of premium fresh-roasted whole-bean coffees. Products include fresh roasted whole-bean single-origin coffee, espresso beans, and drip coffee blends.

GOURMET SPECIALTY FOODS

ChefShop.com
1425 Elliot Avenue West
Seattle, WA 98119
206-286-9988; 800-596-0885
www.chefshop.com

ChefShop.com carries a variety of specialty coffee blends, from an organic dark chocolate 70 percent cocoa to an Ethiopian coffee bar. According to their web site, "The coffee adds a little crunch and a hint of coffee."

COFFEE CANDY AND ICE CREAM

Enjou Chocolat
8 DeHart Street
Morristown, NJ 07960
973-993-9090
www.enjouchocolat.com

A memorable company offering gourmet chocolate, including dark chocolate–covered espresso beans, chocolate coffee bars, and chocolate coffee truffles.

Fran's Chocolates
1325 1st Avenue
Seattle, WA 98101
Mail Order: 800-422-3726; 206-322-0233
www.franschocolates.com

Fran Bigalow's chocolates are made from the finest, freshest, all-natural and, when possible, local and organic ingredients. Chocolates include espresso truffles and dark and milk chocolate.

MarieBelle New York
484 Broome Street
New York, NY 10013
212-431-1768; 212-925-6999
www.mariebelle.com

Coffee chocolate bars, chocolate wafers, and Mocha Hot Chocolate.

Oh! Nuts
888-664-6887
www.ohnuts.com

Premium quality nuts, dried fruit, candy, including a variety of coffee types, and chocolate.

Vosges Haut-Chocolate
Vosges Chicago-Downtown
520 North Michigan Avenue
Chicago, IL 60611
312-644-9450; 888-301-9866
www.vosgeschocolate.com

A prestige chocolate company that provides chocolates paired with coffees.

OLIVE OIL TO PAIR WITH CHOCOLATE

Nick Sciabica & Sons
2150 Yosemite Boulevard
Modesto, CA 95354
800-551-9612
www.sciabica.com

Sciabica specializes in cold-pressed olive oils using several varieties of California olives. Sciabica offers a variety of extra-virgin olive oils.

MORE COFFEE CHAT

Coffee Science Source
www.coffeescience.org

The National Coffee Association's Coffee Science Source is a compendium of news, facts, and figures about the world's favorite beverage.

National Coffee Association of U.S.A., Inc.
45 Broadway
Suite 1140
New York, NY 10006
212-766-4007
www.ncausa.org

The NCA, established in 1911, is the leading trade organization for the coffee industry in the United States. A majority of NCA membership, which accounts for over 90 percent of the U.S. coffee commerce, is comprised of small and mid-sized companies and includes growers, roasters, retailers, import/exporters, wholesaler/suppliers, and allied industry businesses. NCA offers a wide array of services, focusing on market and scientific research, and much more.

Notes

CHAPTER 1:
THE POWER OF COFFEE

1. Oldways Preservation Trust Presents: Refreshingly Good News for Coffee Lovers, Craft Restaurant, New York City, March 22, 2006, "In Praise of Coffee," p. 36.

2. Travis Arndorfer and Kristine Hansen, *The Complete Idiot's Guide to Coffee & Tea* (New York: Alpha Books, 2006), p. 7.

3. Susan Zimmer, *I Love Coffee! Over 100 Easy and Delicious Coffee Drinks* (Kansas City, MO: Andrews McMeel Publishing LLC, pp. 3, 4).

4. Zecuppa Coffee, http://www.zecuppa.com/coffeeterms-bean-grading.htm.

5. Dr. Sanjiv Chopra and Dr. Alan Lotvin, with David Fisher, *Doctor Chopra Says: Medical Facts and Myths Everyone Should Know* (New York: Lotvin, Thomas Dunne Books, 2010), p. 5.

6. Jonny Bowden, Ph.D., *The 150 Healthiest Foods on Earth* (Beverly, Massachusetts: Fair Winds Press, 2007), p. 250.

CHAPTER 2:
AN AWAKENING OF JAVA

1. Oldways Preservation Trust Presents: Refreshingly Good News for Coffee Lovers, Craft Restaurant, New York City, March 22, 2006, "In Praise of Coffee," p. 36.

2. "Innovations That Changed Coffee Culture," *HuffPost Food AOL News*, the Internet newspaper, first posted: March 16, 2011, sponsor-generated content from Starbucks.

3. Coffee Facts—Fun Coffee Information and Trivia, http://gourmet-coffee-zone.com/coffee-facts.html.

4. Courtesy Break Room: The Official Blog of the National Coffee Break: History of Coffee, http://www.nationalcoffeebreak.org/break room/history-of-coffee/.

5. "Innovations That Changed Coffee Culture."

6. Travis Arndorfer and Kristine Hansen, *The Complete Idiot's Guide to Coffee & Tea* (New York: Alpha Books, 2006), p. 7.

7. Coffee Facts—Fun Coffee Information and Trivia, http://gourmet-coffee-zone.com/coffee-facts.html.

8. Ibid.

9. Arndorfer and Hansen, *The Complete Idiot's Guide to Coffee & Tea*, p. 9.

10. Ibid., p. 9.

11. Ibid., p. 9.

12. Arndorfer and Hansen, *The Complete Idiot's Guide to Coffee & Tea*, p. 6.

13. Ibid., p. 7.

14. Ibid., p. 7.

15 Break Room: The Official Blog of the National Coffee Break, History of Coffee, http://www.nationalcoffeebreak.org/breakroom/history-of-coffee/.

16. The Coffee Nazi Brews! The History of Coffee!, http://www.the coffeenazi.com/the-history-of-coffee.

17. Oldways Preservation Trust Presents: Refreshingly Good News for Coffee Lovers, Craft Restaurant, New York City, March 22, 2006, "Coffee Through The Ages," p. 14.

18. Ibid., p. 14.

19. Ibid., p. 14.

20. Ibid., p. 14.

21. Ibid., p. 14.

22. Ibid., p. 14.

23 National Coffee Break, http://www.nationalcoffeebreak.org/new/ history/php.

24. Ibid.

25. Ibid.

Chapter 3:
A Historical Testimony

1. Food Quotes: Coffee, http://www.foodreference.com/html/qcoffee. html.

2. Travis Arndorfer and Kristine Hansen, *The Complete Idiot's Guide to Coffee & Tea* (New York: Alpha Books, 2006), pp. 11–12.

3. www.folgers.com, Explore the Rich Folgers History, http://folgers. com/about-us/folgers-history.aspx.

4. www.eightoclock.com, History/About Us.

5. Coffee Facts—Fun Coffee Information and Trivia, http://gourmet-coffee-zone.com.

6. www.yuban.com, Yuban Story, http://www/yuban.com/yuban/page.

7. www.chockfullonuts.com, History.

8. History of Starbucks, http://www.coffee.org/products/list.

9. www.millstone.com, The Millstone Mission.

10. http://www.mzb-usa.com/history.asp, Massimo Zanetti Beverage USA, Our History.

Chapter 4:
Where Are the Secret Ingredients?

1. Food Quotes: Coffee, http://www.foodreference.com/html/qcoffee/ html.

2. USDA Nutritional Database for Standard Reference, 2010.

3. Jonny Bowden, Ph.D., *The 150 Healthiest Foods on Earth* (Beverly, Massachusetts: Fair Winds Press, 2007), p. 251.

4. Yazheng Liu and David D. Kitts, "Confirmation That the Maillard Reaction Is the Principle Contributor to the Antioxidant Capacity of Coffee Brews," *Food Research International* 44, issue 8 (October 2011): 2418–2424.

5. M. Elena Diaz-Rubio and Fulgencio Saura-Calixto, "Dietary Fiber in Brewed Coffee," *JAgric Food Chemisty* 55 (5) (February 13, 2007): 1990–2003, DOI: 10.1021/jto62839p.

6. Kathleen Thurber, *Midland Reporter-Telegram,* online, "Gourmet Coffee Entrepreneur Works to Add Health Benefits to Morning Ritual," August 3, 2011.

Chapter 5:
Coffee, the New Health Food

1. Food Quotes: Coffee, http://www.foodreference.com/html/qcoffeee.html.

2. Leslie Beck, "Coffee May Prevent Breast Cancer Among Post-menopausal Women," *Globe and Mail* update, p. 1, May 10, 2011, http://www.theglobeandmail.com/life/health/new-health-nutrition/leslie-beck/coffee, retrieved May 19, 2011.

3. Dr. Sanjiv Chopra and Dr. Alan Lotvin, with David Fisher, *Doctor Chopra Says: Medical Facts and Myths Everyone Should Know* (New York: Thomas Dunne Books, St. Martin's Press, New York, New York, 2010), pp. 8–9.

4. Carlotta Galone et al., "Coffee and Tea Intake and Risk of Head and Neck Cancer Epidemiology Consortium," *Cancer Epidemiol Biomarkers Prevention* 19 (July 2010):1723–1736, published online first June 22, 2010, DOI: 10.1158/1055-9965.EPI-10-0191.

5. Kathryn M. Wilson et al., "Coffee Consumption and Prostate Cancer Risk and Progression in the Health Professionals Follow-up," *Journal of the National Cancer Institute*, online May 17, 2011, retrieved May 19, 2011.

6. Masaoki Kawasumiet et al., "Protection from UV-induced Skin Carcinogenesis by Genetic Inhibition of the Ataxia Telangiectasia

and Rad3-retated (ATR) Kinanse," *Proceedings of the National Academy of Sciences*, August 15, 2011, DOI: 10.1073/pnas. 11378108.

7. Jonny Bowden, Ph.D., *The 150 Healthiest Foods on Earth* (Beverly, Massachusetts: Fair Winds Press, 2007), p. 251.

8. Liz Applegate, Ph.D., *101 Miracle Foods That Heal Your Heart* (New York: Prentice Hall Press, 2000), p. 122.

9. Chopra and Lotvin, *Doctor Chopra Says*, p. 5.

CHAPTER 6:
THE MEDITERRANEAN CUPPA COMFORT

1. Oldways Preservation Trust Presents: Refreshingly Good News for Coffee Lovers, Craft Restaurant, New York City, March 22, 2006, p. 37.

2. Used with permission from the Oldways Conference on Refreshingly Good News for Coffee Lovers, New York, 2006, "Coffee and Health," p. 2.

3. Ibid., p. 2.

4. Courtesy Coffee News of Houston, http://www.coffeenewshouston. com/trivia.htm, retrieved May 12, 2011.

CHAPTER 7:
TYPES OF BLENDS AND ROASTS

1. Food Quotes: Coffee, http://www.foodreference.com/html/qcoffee. html.

2. Alpen Sierra Coffee, http://www.alpensierracoffee.com.

CHAPTER 8:
FLAVORED COFFEES

1. Food Quotes, Coffee, http://www.foodreference.com/html/qcoffee. html.

CHAPTER 9:
SWEET MATES

1. Food Quotes: Coffee, http://www.foodreference.com/html/qcoffee.html.
2. Susan Zimmer, *I Love Coffee! Over 100 Easy and Delicious Coffee Drinks* (Kansas City, Missouri: Andrews McMeel, 2007), p. 32.
3. Coffee Facts–Fun Coffee Information and Trivia, http://gourmet-coffee-zone.com/coffee-facts.html.

CHAPTER 10:
THE SKINNY BEVERAGE

1. Food Quotes: Coffee, http://www.foodreference.com/html/qcoffee.html.
2. Ann Louise Gittleman, Edge on Health Blog, The Healing Powers of Coffee, www.annlouise.com/blog/2011/08/02/the-healing-powers-of-coffee.

CHAPTER 11:
ANTIAGING TOAST TO LIFE

1. Coffee Quotes and Sayings About Caffeine, www.quotegarden.com/coffee.html.
2. L. Maia, A. De Mendonca, et al., "Does Caffeine Intake Protect from Alzheimer's Disease?" *European Journal of Neurology*, 9:377–382, DOI: 10.1046/, 1468–1331. 2002.00421.
3. Chuanhai Cao, Li Wang, et al., "Caffeine Synergizes with Another Coffee Component to Increase Plasma GCSF," *Journal of Alzheimer's Disease*, 25(2) (June 28, 2011).
4. G. Webster Ross, M.D., "Association of Coffee and Caffeine Intake with the Risk of Parkinson Disease," *Journal of the American Medical Association* 283 (May 24–31, 2000, © 2000 American Medical Association).
5. Dr. Sanjiv Chopra and Dr. Alan Lotvin, with David Fisher, *Doctor*

Chopra Says: Medical Facts and Myths Everyone Should Know (New York: Thomas Dunne Books, 2010), p. 11.

6. Ibid., p. 11.

7. Used with permission from the Oldways Conference on Refreshingly Good News for Coffee Lovers, New York, 2006.

CHAPTER 12:
HOME REMEDIES FROM YOUR KITCHEN

1. Food Quotes: Coffee, http://www.foodreference.com/html/qcoffee. html.

2. James, "Coffee Cures Baldness, Eases Muscle Pain," http://www.ygoy. com/index.php/coffee-cures-baldness-eases-muscles-pain, published March 20, 2008.

3. "Coffee May Help Prevent Cavities," *American Chemical Society*, March 8, 2002.

4. E. Mattheson, *Annals of Family Medicine* 9 (2011): 299–304, "Tea and Coffee Consumption and MRSA Nasal Carriage."

5. "Cappuccino Coffee Treatment of Xerostomia in Patients Taking Trioyclk Antidepressants, Preliminary Report," *Gdanok Academy of Medicine*, 2002, http://coffeescience.org/retail/Facts.pdf, retrieved July 1, 2011.

6. Used with permission from the Oldways Conference on Refreshingly Good News for Coffee Lovers, New York, 2006, p. 30.

7. "Coffee Cures Gout," http://www.thestar.com (article 217463, published May 25, 2007).

8. Used with permission from the Oldways Conference on Refreshingly Good News for Coffee Lovers, New York, 2006; "Coffee and Brain Health: Coffee and Peak Performance," p. 25.

9. The Editors of FC & A Medical Publishing, Frank W. Cawood and Associates, Inc., *The Folk Remedy Encyclopedia: Olive Oil, Vinegar, Honey and 1,001 Other Home Remedies* (Peachtree City, Georgia: FC & A Medical Publishing, 2004), p. 220.

10. "Little Known Facts About Coffee: Effect of Breakfast and Caf-

feine on Performance and Mood in the Late Morning and After Lunch," *Neuropsychobiology:* 1992, http://coffeescience.org/retail/Facts.pdf, retrieved September 13, 2011.

11. *Neuropsychobiology* 1192, http://coffeescience.org/retail/Facts.pdf, retrieved July 1, 2011; James, "Coffee Cures Baldness," www.ygoy.com/index.php/coffee-cures-baldness-eases-muscle-pain, retrieved July 4, 2011.

12. "The Effect of Caffeine on Handwriting Movements in Skilled Writers," *Hum MovSci*, 2006, http://coffeescience.org/retail/Facts pdf, retrieved July 1, 2011.

13. "Little Known Facts About Coffee. Low-Dose Repeated Caffeine Administration for Circadian-Phase-Dependent Performance Degradation During Extended Wakefulness," *Sleep*, 2004, http://coffeescience.org/retail/Facts.pdf, retrieved September 13, 2011.

CHAPTER 13:
COFFEE CRAZE: GROUNDS FOR THE HOUSEHOLD

1. Oldways Preservation Trust Presents: Refreshingly Good News for Coffee Lovers, Craft Restaurant, New York City, March 22, 2006, p. 36.

CHAPTER 14:
THE BEAUTY OF COFFEE

1. Food Quotes: Coffee, http://www.foodreference.com/html/qcoffee.html.

CHAPTER 15:
SPECIALTY COFFEE CONNOISSEURS

1. Food Quotes: Coffee, http://www.foodreference.com/html/qcoffee.html.

2. Alpen Sierra Coffee Company, http://www.alpensierracoffee.com/About/c2/p8/History/pages/html.

3. Alpen Sierra Coffee Company, http://www.alpensierracoffee.com/blog.php.

4. Coffees of Hawaii, www.coffeesofhawaii.com/company/history.

5. Coffee.org, www.coffee.org, About Us, the Coffee.org Team.

6. Coffee, Tea & Spice, www.coffeecoffee.com. Welcome to Coffee, Tea & Spice.

7. White Coffee Company, www.whitecoffee.com/about us.htm, Our History—White Coffee.

CHAPTER 16:
COFFEE IS NOT HOT FOR EVERYONE

1. Food Quotes: Coffee, http://www.foodreference.com/html/qcoffee.html.

2. Bonnie Edwards, R.N., *America's Favorite Drug: Coffee and Your Health* (Berkeley, California: Odian Press, 1992), pp. 9–10.

3. Ibid., pp. 33–34.

4. Ibid., pp. 45–46.

5. Interstitial Cystitis Network, http://www.icnsales.com/coffee-low-acid/.

6. Edwards, *America's Favorite Drug*, p. 92.

7. Ibid., pp. 93–94.

CHAPTER 17:
THE JOY OF COOKING WITH COFFEE

1. Oldways Preservation Trust Presents: Refreshingly Good News for Coffee Lovers, Craft Restaurant, New York, March 22, 2006, p. 36.

CHAPTER 18:
HERE COMES THE COFFEE

1. Think Exist Quotes, http://thinkexist.com/quotation/only_irish_coffee_provides_in_a_single_glass_all/166275.html.

2. Food Quotes: Coffee, http://www.foodreference.com/html/qcoffee html.

Selected Bibliography

Andorfer, Travis, and Kristine Hansen. *The Complete Idiot's Guide to Coffee & Tea.* New York: Alpha Books, 2006.

Bowden, Jonny, Ph.D., C.N.S. *The 150 Healthiest Foods on Earth: The Surprising, Unbiased Truth About What You Should Eat and Why.* Beverly, MA: Fair Winds Press, 2007.

Chopra, Dr. Sanjiv, and Dr. Alan Lotvin, with David Fisher. *Doctor Chopra Says: Medical Facts and Myths Everyone Should Know.* New York: St. Martin's Press, 2010.

Kummer, Corby. *The Joy of Coffee: The Essential Guide to Buying, Brewing, and Enjoying,* revised and updated. New York: Houghton Mifflin Company, 2003.

Pendergrast, Mark. *Uncommon Grounds: The History of Coffee and How It Transformed Our World.* Revised Edition. New York: Basic Books, 2010.

Sciabica, Gemma Sanita. *Baking Sensational Sweets with California Olive Oil.* Modesto, CA: Gemma Sanita Sciabica, 2005.

Sciabica, Gemma Sanita. *Baking with California Olive Oil: Dolci and Biscotti Recipes.* Modesto, CA: Gemma Sanita Sciabica, 2002.

Sciabica, Gemma Sanita. *Cooking with California Olive Oil: Popular Recipes.* Modesto, CA: Gemma Sanita Sciabica, 2001.

Sciabica, Gemma Sanita. *Cooking with California Olive Oil: Recipes from the Heart for the Heart.* Modesto, CA: Gemma Sanita Sciabica, 2009.

Sciabica, Gemma Sanita. *Cooking with California Olive Oil: Treasured Family Recipes.* Modesto, CA: Gemma Sanita Sciabica, 1998.

Zimmer, Susan. *I Love Coffee! Over 100 Easy and Delicious Coffee Drinks.* Kansas City, MO: Andrews McMeel, 2007.